Managing Diversity in Health Care

Managing Diversity in Health Care

Lee Gardenswartz
Anita Rowe

Jossey-Bass Publishers • San Francisco

Substantial discounts on bulk quantities of Jossey-Bass books are available to corporations, professional associations, and other organizations. For details and discount information, contact the special sales department at Jossey-Bass Inc., Publishers (415) 433–1740; Fax (800) 605–2665.

For sales outside the United States, please contact your local Simon & Schuster International Office.

Jossey-Bass Web address: http://www.josseybass.com

 Manufactured in the United States of America on Lyons Falls Turin Book. This paper is acid-free and 100 percent totally chlorine-free.

Library of Congress Cataloging-in-Publication Data

Gardenswartz, Lee.
    Managing diversity in health care/Lee Gardenswartz. Anita Rowe.
—1st ed.
      p. cm.
    Includes bibliographical references and index.
    ISBN 0-7879-4041-0 (alk. paper)
      1. Transcultural medical care—United States. 2. Minorities—
Medical care—United States. 3. Minorities—Health and hygiene—
United States. I. Rowe, Anita. II. Title.
RA418.5.T73.G37 1998
362.1'089'00973—dc21   98-14745
                                                                CIP

FIRST EDITION
HB Printing   10 9 8 7 6 5 4 3 2

Contents

Acknowledgments

We would like to thank the many colleagues and clients who have generously shared their knowledge and experience with us. In particular, we would like to give a special thanks to the following people:

- Debby Crossland and the Sisters of Providence Health System staff at Yakima/Toppenish Central Washington Service Area
- Elizabeth Wu and her colleagues at Kaiser Permanente
- Kurt Miyamoto and Paul Czajka at Little Company of Mary Hospital
- Harriet Glass Ulmer and the staff at LA Care
- Howard Horwitz and Wes Curry at the American College of Physician Executives
- Andy Pasternack, our editor, for his painstaking and meticulous revisions and gracious feedback
- Ron Matheson for his astute suggestions and the cheerful, competent, and steadfast manner in which he made the many revisions that culminated in the final manuscript

The Authors

LEE GARDENSWARTZ is a native of Denver and a graduate of the University of Colorado at Boulder. ANITA ROWE is a native of Los Angeles and a graduate of the University of California Los Angeles. Each worked as a secondary teacher and staff development facilitator in the Los Angeles Unified School District for a number of years before returning to academia to earn a Doctorate of Human Behavior from the United States International University in 1981.

Gardenswartz and Rowe began helping organizations with diversity in 1977 while working with the Los Angeles Unified School District to deal with its diversity challenges at the time of mandatory integration. Since that time they have specialized in the "human side of management," working with a variety of regional and national clients—including GTE, Southern California Gas Company, the IRS, the Society of Consumer Affairs Professionals, DWP, The Los Angeles Times, FHP, the State of California Department of Health Services, British Telecommunications, UCLA, South Coast AQMD, First State Bank, VA Medical Center, MCA, and The Prudential—helping them to manage change, handle stress, build productive and cohesive work teams, and create inter-cultural understanding and harmony in the workplace. In addition, they have helped organizations through their writing on diversity. Their book *Managing Diversity: A Complete Desk Reference and Planning Guide* (1993), which won the book-of-the-year award from the

Society for Human Resource Managers in 1994, has served as a primary guide to organizations in structuring their diversity initiatives, providing not only conceptual information but also techniques and tools. They write a regular column in *Managing Diversity* newsletter; have written articles on diversity for publications such as *Physician Executive, College and University Personnel Journal,* and *Working World;* and have been featured in *Personnel Journal.* They have also coauthored the *Managing Diversity Survival Guide* (1994), *The Diversity Tool Kit* (1994), and *Diverse Teams at Work* (1995).

Gardenswartz and Rowe have lectured widely, giving keynote speeches, facilitating team-building retreats, and teaching seminars across the country. They have made guest appearances on such programs as *Mid-Morning LA,* CNN's *News Night, Sun Up San Diego, AM Northwest, Crier and Company,* and *The Michael Jackson Show.* They also teach about diversity through institutions such as the National Multicultural Institute in Washington, D.C., and the Intercultural Communication Institute in Portland, Oregon.

Introduction

- Twenty percent of physicians practicing in the United States are foreign trained.[1]

- Minorities are the majority in six of the eight largest urban areas in the United States, as well as in two thousand other communities across the country.[2]

- In the Los Angeles area, 42 percent of the population speaks a language other than English at home.

- Medi-Cal Managed Care, the state of California's equivalent to the Medicare system, now requires health care providers to give "culturally appropriate" and "linguistically competent" services.[3]

Welcome to the complexities of twenty-first century medicine. Although health care has been in the vortex of revolutionary change for the last two decades, change continues to come at a relentless pace. From the advent of diagnostic-related groupings (DRGs) in the early 1980s to the proliferation of health maintenance organizations (HMOs) and managed care systems of the 1990s, transitions in the industry have been fundamental and challenging. The current sociological transformation brought about by increasingly complicated and pluralistic demographics in communities from coast to coast may be even more sweeping, and more pregnant with both obstacles and opportunities, than previous upheavals have been.

In hospitals around the country, staff, physicians, and patients of different cultures, backgrounds, and values come together to heal, to seek and offer comfort, and to save lives. In the multicultural meeting place that is an increasing reality in most health care institutions, health care staff and those they serve often speak different languages, operate according to different norms, and experience misunderstanding and discord that can impair care.

In such an environment, health care institutions need to give staff the information and tools that will enable them to work effectively with diverse colleagues and provide quality care to a wider and wider range of patients. This book offers health care professionals a road map for creating inclusive environments that attract open-minded staff who seek continuous learning as a way to enhance cooperative relationships with both diverse coworkers and diverse patients. It also provides practical information and activities to equip staff at all levels, from executives to direct care providers, with the awareness, knowledge, and skills to give effective care to patients—care that involves a variety of worldviews about life and death, rituals and practices for healing, and norms and definitions about what constitutes good health care delivery. Finally, this book is written for health care providers in the United States who are trying to integrate a wide variety of acceptable practices into their repertoire of skills. When all is said and done, adaptability, knowledge, and openness can provide a critical difference in offering a positive health care experience. Juggling the multiple and varied expectations of the wide array of patients who walk through your doors is, to say the very least, challenging and potentially frustrating. It is in the high-anxiety clinical environment that patients are often most needy and vulnerable. Meshing the assumptions and expectations of the many caregivers who are part of a patient's experience with the assumptions and expectations of the patient and family who need treatment, understanding, respect, and sensitivity is what this book is about. True healing requires not only the correcting of a disease or the abatement of pain, but also the creation of a condition of wholeness—psychological, physical, and emotional well-being. We believe that the following chapters show the way toward achieving that wholeness.

Wholeness and Well-Being: In the Eye of the Beholder

More than a hundred years ago Nathaniel Hawthorne observed something that makes infinite sense about health care today. "He deemed it essential, it would seem, to know the man before attempting to do him good."[4] This book is our attempt to help you know not only the man or the woman but, in fact, the whole family so that you can do good for all with whom you come in contact.

It is legitimate for you as a health care practitioner to wonder what a condition of wholeness and well-being might entail when applied to health care and diversity. To begin with, any effective diversity education has the teaching of different cultural practices as a critical component. Staff learn about the wide array of norms and rituals related to such universals as life, death, marriage, and healing. The answer to the question of what constitutes healing and well-being is: it depends. Employees learn that care and healing lie in the eye of the beholder, and that this eye is powerfully under the influence of culture. There are a variety of ways to achieve well-being, and certainly one component of diversity knowledge means understanding the development and various definitions of treatment and healing.

"Over time, healing has been accomplished by dancing, praying, giving offerings to gods, going to certain places, administering different substances, and even by more radical methods of cutting into the body or removing certain body parts. Health, disease, and death reach different levels of acceptance in different cultures. Religious beliefs, social structure, and the environment around us modulate the way we live and look. They also mandate the degree of intervention of invasiveness allowed into the human body."[5] This quote by Suzanne Salimbene, intercultural communication expert, and Jack W. Graczykowski, a physician, only begins to indicate the enormous differences possible in definitions of appropriate treatment. For societies and people steeped in the use of the supernatural to aid healing, high-tech medicine does not seem to be all that it is cracked up to be. The role of both science and the supernatural in the healing process may be worth a substantial discussion as you try to understand your patient base. So might the extent to which extraordinary measures should be extended or to which surgery should be identified as a beneficial intervention.

Understanding how medicine has evolved and changed is only part of the content of this book. We would also like to increase the reader's awareness and understanding of the significance of culture as a shaper of participation in health care treatment. Culture deeply influences a person's view of life and death, his or her expectations about what constitutes a desirable doctor-patient relationship, and his or her perceptions of excellence related to standards of care in traditional Western medicine. It also involves views of alternative therapies that do not include Western medicine at all.

A research team at the University of Southern California completed a study in 1995 that shows the profound influence of culture on such basic medical assumptions as the right to die and the control of one's medical destiny. The study drew on interviews with Los Angeles County residents, all sixty-five or older, from four different groups. The data indicated that 45 percent of Korean Americans and 65 percent of Mexican Americans would not want to be told if they had a fatal illness, and both groups generally expected their family members to make treatment decisions for them if they were gravely ill.[6] What impact might these preferences have on the behavior of doctors schooled in American medical norms, which value telling patients the full story so that individuals can exercise autonomy in their treatment decisions? In contrast, nearly 90 percent of blacks and whites want the unvarnished truth when the prognosis is delivered. In keeping with American cultural norms, these patients do not want to burden their families with painful, wrenching medical decisions. Rather, they prefer to express therapeutic wishes in advance through the use of documents such as living wills. Any physician practicing at an urban medical center will likely encounter all this variety, and then some, in patient preferences. Thus, general awareness of beliefs, values, behaviors, and preferences among a wide variety of patients—both citizen and noncitizen, those here for generations and the newly immigrated—is part of the conceptual information an effective health care practitioner needs in this day and age. That information is in this book.

We do not offer specific rules and practices for any particular cultural group, as though such rules and practices could be gospel that makes behavior predictable. The body of knowledge about culture and ethnicity is not formulaic. It is not our desire to reinforce stereotypes, and we know that within any group there is considerable variation. We do present information documented from previous studies and the general experience of health care professionals. We offer for your consideration patterns and generalities based on observations, and literature from theorists and practitioners who are well versed in their fields. Once you have learned this information, it can aid you in understanding patients' behavior, attitudes, and choices.

In addition to shedding light on some general cultural patterns, values, and beliefs, we also want to emphasize that there are differences between individuals within a culture as well as differences between, for example, various Hispanic groups, such as Cubans, Mexicans, and Puerto Ricans. There are also alternatives in treatment and values between Western and non-Western medical practices.

It seems, then, that what is called for is enough information about the various dimensions of health care treatment shaped by culture to open the eyes of all health care practitioners, and enough culture-specific information to help health care providers respond in a way that allows patients' needs to be met. *Cultural flexibility* is the best approach. By gaining both general and specific information about the intersection between health care delivery and culture, a larger repertoire of treatments and interventions will be available to you. Armed with this knowledge, it is possible for all health care practitioners to serve patients and their families better and more sensitively. In addition, people in the health care field should be able to understand and interact more effectively with colleagues who undoubtedly will also have been influenced by a variety of explicit and implicit cultural norms.

This book is also designed to help the reader wrestle with complex questions that defy easy answers. In addition to the obvious questions, such as What is excellent care? and Whose definition of care is accurate? a series of relevant, thorny questions need to be considered from the highest strategic levels of the organization down to the operational levels of staff who most directly interface with patients. For example

- It would no doubt be difficult for a Western-trained physician who had been taught the importance of a doctor-patient partnership to respond to patients who prefer a decisive, autocratic medical opinion rather than a collegial discussion of options. This situation becomes more complicated when the partnership-oriented physician perceives that he or she loses the status and credibility of being an expert simply by engaging the patient in discussion about treatment.

- After being reared in a society that for the last thirty years has fought for strong women's rights, culminating in a woman's right to choose whether to carry a pregnancy to term, how should a physician respond when he interacts with cultures in which key medical decisions for women are often made by males in positions of authority in the family, and infrequently by the woman herself?

- What is an appropriate physician response when a Chinese patient needs surgery but may be opposed to it because Confucius says that "only those who shall be truly revered are those who at the end of their lives will return their bodies whole and sound"?[7]

- What is the criteria for sensitive and appropriate nurse behavior when an entire extended family wants to come and stay with a patient as a means of indicating love and support but the hospital rules allow for only two visitors, not twenty-five?

These are just a few of the conundrums that present substantial challenges as the U.S. medical system deals with growing cultural complexity. To help you engage in these and other multifaceted issues, *Managing Diversity in Health Care* is organized to increase your understanding of culture, diversity, stereotypes, and expectations at the level of the individual first.

Culture and ethnicity are certainly important considerations when examining the current health care delivery system, but they are by no means all of the diversities that are seen. Socioeconomic level also plays a huge role in caregivers' assumptions about and expectations of their patients. Many doctors, for example, appear to be more comfortable and willing to exchange information with patients of a high socioeconomic status. The more patients are like their doctors economically, the more the patients and doctors understand each other and the less confusion and misunderstanding there are.[8] Other diversity-related factors that shape perceptions include the age of patients, their level of education, their geographic region, and their religious beliefs and practices. All human beings have biases, preferences, and assumptions, some subtle, some not. Health care professionals cannot be expected to be more human, or humane, than the rest of the population, but understanding predictable knee-jerk biases is critical to effective interactions on the job.

Organization of the Contents

To help practitioners get beyond these biases and assumptions, and to help all caregivers deliver a culturally appropriate standard of care, we have organized this book to help readers become conscious of their own assumptions. The book will help you to look not only at caregiver-to-patient relationships but also at staff-to-staff interactions. Finally, we look at leader effectiveness in the current rapidly changing environment. What decisions are made at the executive levels that reward cultural flexibility and sensitivity? How are staff at all levels held accountable for being culturally competent? What barriers to open and responsive care exist, and what systems need to be created or refined to foster culturally competent care?

To help you learn at both the intrapersonal and interpersonal levels, and to guide you in assessing and eliminating any systems obstacles that may inhibit healing, we provide the following chapters:

1. "Why Diversity Is Good for Business: Marketplace and Workforce Issues" looks at population and demographic shifts. In addition to acknowledging the changing face of America, we explore the challenges and opportunities presented by this pluralistic patient base.

2. "The Dimensions of Health Care Diversity" defines the four layers of diversity and looks at the impact that each of the dimensions within these layers has on staff relationships and on relationships with patients, families, and visitors.

3. "The Truth About Cultural Programming" focuses on the pervasive role of ethnicity in shaping attitudes, needs, and beliefs about health care, and on the influence of theses attitudes, needs, and beliefs on interactions, treatments, rituals, and norms. The chapter also highlights some of the values, dilemmas, and conflicts, and cites examples of variation in norms and preferences as well as misunderstandings that are often present in a cross-cultural environment.

4. "Achieving Practical Cultural Literacy" builds on the cross-cultural knowledge presented in Chapter Three and offers concrete examples of the differences that culture makes in providing care to pluralistic patients. It identifies factors that influence a person's

level of acculturation, and it focuses on some specific cultural factors that shape the health care experience, including standards of privacy, the importance and criteria of status, and beliefs about the body, healing, and dying.

5. "Improving Communication in Diverse Environments" also builds on the knowledge and awareness of cross-cultural differences gained in Chapter Three by focusing on one specific dimension of culture—communication—and looking at relevant topics such as giving and getting feedback, communicating with the help of interpreters and translators, and soliciting relevant information in culturally sensitive ways.

6. "Removing Stereotypes That Block High-Quality Care" explores the subtle assumptions, expectations, and biases that hinder care and service. These stereotypes are explored not only intrapersonally but also systemwide. Are there institutional biases that minimize promotional opportunities for some people? Do certain patients get a little more effort expended on their behalf? Confronting the subtle and unconscious assumptions that all human beings make is the first step toward minimizing the negative impact of those assumptions.

7. "The Diversity Leadership Challenge" identifies qualities of effective leaders and executives who are responsible for and effective in bringing about real culture change. The focus is on accountability, role-modeling, walking the talk, and changing the norms so that the organization of the future has the vision to reward the kind of behaviors and knowledge necessary to create cutting-edge health care. Ethics are also discussed.

8. "Overcoming Barriers to Change" targets some specific arenas for change if an organization is truly committed to removing obstacles to diversity. By looking at individual attitudes and awareness, managerial skills, and organizational policies and practices, real change becomes concrete and doable. To enhance specificity even more, we provide seven steps that are essential for consideration in any long-term change process.

9. "Creative Organizational Problem Solving" presents real, complex examples of health-care-related dilemmas that illustrate the various challenges and in-progress solutions currently being utilized by several different health care organizations.

Finally, a lengthy and current resources section provides staff with diversity-related resources of all types, including annotated lists of pertinent books, videos, articles, newsletters, and published training materials. It also enumerates specific health care resources.

How to Use This Book

There are a number of ways to use this book. It can be read straight through for a thorough overview of critical concepts and information. The reader can also target specific sections to gain answers to particular questions or information about a specific issue. In addition, the models and checklists can be used as assessment and training tools. For those who need training resources, a companion trainer's guide containing approximately forty reproducible activities and worksheets will soon be available. These activities reinforce the lessons learned from the book and help staff to increase awareness, gain knowledge, and develop skills to grapple with the complex dilemmas sometimes encountered in a diverse health care environment.

This practical book attempts to help busy health care professionals who are trying to do more with less to help patients and families experience emotional and physical healing. With that utopian goal in mind, we reiterate that the book is written for those who design and implement an organization's strategic vision. It is equally appropriate for those who train and develop staff to meet the goals of that strategy, as well as for direct caregivers. It provides a solid body of information about various aspects of diversity and their influence on health care practices. Although conceptual information is a critical first step in learning, learning activities are also provided to help readers who are trying to increase their competence in dealing with diversity. Administrators, directors of education and staff development, trainers, managers, and supervisors will find relevant, on-target information and tools to make diversity a competitive advantage.

This book is both a call to and a plan for action. Enjoy!

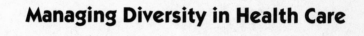

Managing Diversity in Health Care

1

Why Diversity Is Good for Business

Marketplace and Workforce Issues

- "Latinos and Asians will account for more than half the growth in the U.S. population every year for the next half century and beyond."[1]
- "More than 100 languages are spoken in the school systems of New York City, Chicago, Los Angeles, and Fairfax County, Virginia."[2]

With salsa overtaking ketchup as the top-selling condiment and Spanish radio stations at the top of the charts in cities such as San Antonio and Los Angeles, the abstract statistics about these changes begin to become more concrete.

Demographic Changes: An Increasingly Complex Patient and Employee Base

America has always been a nation of immigrants, and the overwhelming majority of Americans claim ancestry from another continent. The current pattern of immigration is different, however, from that of the early 1900s, which witnessed the century's other great wave of newcomers. At the beginning of the twentieth century and through the first five decades, the majority of immigrants were Europeans; the more recent picture is a very different one. In the last thirty years, revolutions, wars, and economic crises around the world have brought people of widely different backgrounds, languages, and cultures to the United States. Although in 1940 70 percent of immigrants came from Europe, in 1992 only 15 percent did. The rest came from Asia (37 percent) and from Latin America and the Caribbean (44 percent).[3] Today's settlers bring a wide array of native languages as well as cultural norms and religions. Los Angeles, a city where more than 30 percent of the population is nonnative English speakers and where Buddhists and Muslims outnumber many Christian denominations, is perhaps a harbinger of the change that can be expected across the country.

According to multicultural marketing expert Marlene Rossman, "nearly one of every four Americans claims African, Asian, Hispanic, or American Indian ancestry, compared to only one in five in the 1980 census. The rate of increase in the minority population between 1980 and 1990 was nearly twice the rate of increase between 1970 and 1980."[4] Although the Census Bureau acknowledges that some of the minority population gets lost in the counting, and that the number of individuals of mixed race is growing, the current snapshot of the U.S. population shows that

- Blacks number 30 million (about 12 percent of the population).
- Hispanics currently number 22.4 million (9 percent), but they will soon be the largest minority in the country.
- 7.3 million people are Asians (3 percent), and 2 million are American Indians (0.8 percent).[5]

In such a pluralistic environment, the word *minority* is inaccurate. According to an Associated Press article, racial and ethnic minorities—identified as blacks, Asians, Latinos, Pacific Islanders, American Indians, Eskimos, and Aleuts—are the majority in thousands of communities around the country. As we have already noted, racial minorities are the majority in six of the eight U.S. cities that have a population of more than one million people. Detroit is 80 percent minority; the other five cities are Los Angeles,

Chicago, New York, Houston, and Dallas. Not only large urban areas are undergoing demographic transformation, however. One hundred eighty-six counties and 1,930 cities, towns, and other municipalities are also dominated demographically by racial and ethnic minorities.[6]

Not all areas of the country are equally affected by these changes. California, Texas, Florida, Illinois, and New Jersey are home to three out of four new immigrants. Los Angeles has the largest population of Mexicans, Filipinos, Salvadorans, and Koreans outside of their home countries of any city in the world, with additional large enclaves of Iranians, Chinese, Armenians, Native Americans, Pacific Islanders, and Ethiopians. New York has significant percentages of Puerto Ricans, Dominicans, Chinese, and Koreans. Each area of the country has its own uniquely changing pattern of newcomers and established populations. What is more, individuals from these increasingly varied backgrounds constitute the workforce in today's health care institutions, making the workplace at hospitals, clinics, and health care providing agencies truly international in composition.

When the numbers are this attention getting, and when the meaning of the words *minority* and *majority* are inverted, it is time for health care providers to wonder: Who are our patients, and what are their needs? How can we serve them effectively? How are these demographic changes shown on our staff? What must our institution do differently to deal with these changes? What do these latest statistics mean for our traditional outreach? For visionaries open to change, this demographic shift is the half-full glass.

Consider the changing demographics of your patient population and your workforce. Knowing the information outlined in Exhibits 1.1 and 1.2 about your patient and your employee base is a first step in answering these questions. When you fill out the demographic sheets in the exhibits, notice not only the information you have about your patients and staff but also the information you do not have. Consider what direction your analysis suggests. For example, a match between patients and workforce may mean greater understanding of patients' needs, while a disparity between the two may indicate a need for interpreters or intercultural communication training. Staff who speak a variety of native languages may point to a need for the kind of training that one government agency provides to help employees develop a multilingual ear. If more information is needed about the population in your service area, a task force may be called for to design ways to obtain it. If there is a need to learn about the health care needs and cultures of people who are part of a particular ethnic or religious group, who speak a certain language, or who live within certain economic constraints, more cultural diversity training may be indicated. If employees' beliefs and attitudes might unconsciously interfere with their giving the best care to or working productively with people of other groups, sensitivity training might be recommended.

What These Population Shifts Mean to Health Care

In many areas of the country, the reality of health care is increasingly similar to Cigna's Grand Avenue Health Center in downtown Los Angeles, located near significant Latino, African American, and Asian communities. Not only is the patient population diverse, but the workforce is as well. Thirty-five percent of the staff is Latino, 20 percent is Filipino, 5 percent is Thai, and the remainder is Euro-American or Korean. Many employees now speak Spanish, and the center makes it a priority to hire bilingual staff.[7]

As the largest contractor providing health care to MediCal recipients, Cigna serves many patients who are poor (earning less than $750 a month for a family of two). In addition, this center serves an increasing immigrant population that brings different cultural expectations about health care, which at times come into conflict with traditional U.S. medical practices. Folk remedies and healers may sometimes be preferred by patients. Different patterns of disease may be seen—for example, a reemergence of tuberculosis as a serious health problem and higher rates of diabetes among

EXHIBIT 1.1 Changing Demographics: Do You Know Your Patients?

General Information:

Household Income

| | Under $20,000 | _____ | $20,000–$35,000 | _____ |
| | $35,000–$50,000 | _____ | Over $50,000 | _____ |

Age   20–35 _____   36–49 _____   50+ _____

Gender   Male _____   Female _____

Married   _____

Single   _____

Married with children _____   Average number of children _____

Single-parent family   _____   Average number of children _____

Ethnic Groups

African American	_____	Latino	_____
Filipino	_____	Korean	_____
Armenian	_____	Chinese	_____
Indian	_____	Japanese	_____
Middle Eastern	_____	Russian	_____
Native American	_____	Euro-American	_____
Vietnamese	_____	Lao	_____
Cambodian	_____	Haitian	_____
Other	_____		

Education Level

Elementary school	_____	Some high school	_____
High school diploma	_____	Some college	_____
Graduated college	_____	Advanced degree	_____

Languages Spoken

English	_____	Spanish	_____	Russian	_____
Korean	_____	Tagalog	_____	Mandarin	_____
Vietnamese	_____	French	_____	Cantonese	_____
Cambodian	_____	Laotian	_____	Farsi	_____
Other	_____				

Bilingual _____   Limited or non-English speaking _____

EXHIBIT 1.2   Changing Demographics: Do You Know Your Workforce?

General Information:

Household Income

| Under $20,000 _____ $20,000–$35,000 _____
            $35,000–$50,000 _____   Over $50,000   _____

Age   20–35 _____   36–49 _____   50+ _____

Gender   Male _____   Female _____

Married   _____

Single   _____

Married with children _____   Average number of children _____

Single-parent family   _____   Average number of children _____

Ethnic Groups

African American	_____	Latino	_____
Filipino	_____	Korean	_____
Armenian	_____	Chinese	_____
Indian	_____	Japanese	_____
Middle Eastern	_____	Russian	_____
Native American	_____	Euro-American	_____
Vietnamese	_____	Lao	_____
Cambodian	_____	Haitian	_____
Other	_____		

Education Level

Elementary school	_____	Some high school	_____
High school diploma	_____	Some college	_____
Graduated college	_____	Advanced degree	_____

Languages Spoken

English	_____	Spanish	_____	Russian	_____
Korean	_____	Tagalog	_____	Mandarin	_____
Vietnamese	_____	French	_____	Cantonese	_____
Cambodian	_____	Laotian	_____	Farsi	_____
Other	_____				

Bilingual _____   Limited or non-English speaking _____

some Latino men. In addition, changes in the use of services are seen, with increased use of emergency rooms (ERs) by immigrant patients.[8]

Population shifts such as those faced at the Grand Avenue Clinic are not only having an impact on the relationship between provider and patient, they are also influencing relationships among staff. What happens when physicians and licensed staff are trained in different parts of the world, under different medical systems? How do staff members speaking a variety of native languages communicate effectively, especially in the high-pressure, fast-paced world of health care, where clear communication is critical and misunderstandings can cause irreparable damage?

Meeting New Contractor and Managed Care Requirements

What is required of health care providers is vastly different from what was required in the days when patient, physician, nurse, and other hospital personnel all came from similar backgrounds, spoke the same language, and shared a set of expectations and assumptions about health care. For example, a patient raised in the United States might want to be given all the facts, including the bad news about a diagnosis, while an Asian patient might prefer a vague explanation, viewing the mere mention of a terminal illness as a death sentence that upsets inner harmony and hastens the progression of the disease. A patient who was bred in America might have more confidence in a physician who runs many tests so she can give a more accurate diagnosis, while an immigrant patient may feel insecure with a doctor who cannot diagnose on the spot. An American patient might expect to ask many questions and make health care decisions himself, while a Latino patient might expect the physician, nurse, or therapist to be the expert and take charge, and an Asian patient might want the whole family involved in health care choices.

In addition to the disparities in behavioral preferences that may be present, there are very real language and educational differences that can hinder communication. For instance, nonnative English-speaking individuals often nod and respond that they understand directions, then proceed to take incorrect action. One Southeast Asian couple were distressed when their child's ear infection was not improving. The physician had given explicit directions in how to use the medication and the parents had nodded vigorously when asked if they understood. However, upon investigation the physician discovered that they had been putting the medication in the child's ear (giving it aurally) instead of having him swallow it (giving it orally).

To help overcome these obstacles, some managed care plans require providers contracting with them to offer culturally and linguistically competent care. According to intercultural expert and author Suzanne Salimbene, "'culturally appropriate' means the capacity of individuals or organizations to effectively identify the health practices and behaviors of target populations; to design programs, interventions, and services which effectively address cultural and language barriers to the delivery of appropriate and necessary health services, and to evaluate and contribute to the on-going improvement of those efforts."[9]

In what might be an indication of future requirements across the country, the State of California's Department of Health Services has drafted the Cultural Index of Accessibility to Care (see Exhibit 1.3). Other states may have, or may be planning, similar guidelines.

Analyzing the Challenges and Opportunities That Diversity Brings

All change cuts two ways, and increasing diversity in the world of health care is certainly a case in point. The obstacles may be more apparent initially, because language barriers, conflicting health care practices, or cultural differences that have an impact

EXHIBIT 1.3 State of California, Department of Health Services, Cultural Index of Accessibility to Care.

Cultural Index of Accessibility to Care. When an ethnic group with limited English language capability is five percent (or more) in a postal zone of a managed care contractor's enrollment (and the contractor's total Medi-Cal enrollment is 1,000 or more), the following services are required:

Plan Coverage Information. Information about membership in the managed care plan, including details about coverage, shall be presented in the languages of the members, both orally and in writing, as specified above. Plan member services departments should have the resources, including staff persons, to go to the community centers and other locations where their enrollees gather to ensure that their members know how their plan works and how to use it, and to identify and solve individual access problems. Plans which distribute informational literature as part of their outreach efforts shall ensure that it is culturally appropriate. Individual plans shall have the flexibility to decide the extent to which such outreach arrangements are necessary to meet their members' needs. The plan membership process also must have the ability to include in plan records information about a non-English speaking member's primary language.

Health Education Programs. Managed care plans also must design health education programs which are culturally appropriate for their members. The health education efforts, which will complement local public health activities, must be designed using community-based needs assessments and other relevant information available from State and local governmental agencies and community groups. Educational programs must make use of health promotion approaches and health informational literature which recognize enrolled groups' values and health beliefs.

Health Care Provider Orientation and Training. Managed care provider orientation and training programs must include components designed to facilitate communication with non-English speaking patients and patients who don't hold mainstream health beliefs. Specifically, this module should provide the plan's direct care givers the following:

1. Orientation to the effective use of non-medically trained translators to take patient histories and to assist with other communication related to treating the patient;

2. Strategies for using the belief patterns and family support systems of the patients to promote adherence to the course of treatment as well as assumption of personal responsibility for preventive health behaviors;

3. Background information for identifying and treating certain diseases and health conditions not commonly found in the dominant population.

Qualification of Translators. Managed care plans must assure and be prepared to demonstrate the competence of their staff who are responsible for translation services for plan members. Such competence must include the ability to translate commonly used primary care medical terms from English to languages used by the plan members.

Appointments and Medical Advice. Managed care plans must have bilingual or multilingual personnel staffing their medical advice and appointment systems. The training of these staff persons must enhance their understanding of the difficulties members who have been used to FFS (fee for service) arrangements might have in learning to use managed care systems. In addition, discharge planners must be able to provide linguistically and culturally appropriate information to ensure that patients understand and are willing to follow their post-treatment instructions.

Member Satisfaction. Annual surveys that assess members' satisfaction with the plan and their coverage must be an integral feature of the Medi-Cal managed care program. These surveys must be designed to accommodate language and culture differences among members.

Source: California Department of Health Services, *Expanding Medi-Cal Managed Care* (Sacramento: California Department of Health Services, 1994).

on communication can present frustrating hindrances to productive relationships and effective care.

There are some exciting potential benefits for health care professions and organizations, however. Physicians, nurses, therapists, and technicians often report feeling enriched, enlightened, and empowered when they begin to communicate in another language, learn about other cultures, or form bonds with colleagues and patients of different backgrounds. As one physician, Elizabeth Gutrecht, a bilingual and bicultural obstetrician and gynecologist who has made a career of treating Spanish-speaking and immigrant patients, says, "I enjoy . . . working with the elderly Hispanic ladies especially because there aren't a lot of doctors who understand their concerns and who can speak to them. I don't feel that my role as a doctor is to impose my views on them, but to help them take care of themselves."[10]

There are also financial benefits to hospitals that capitalize on the opportunities presented by diversity. For example, one urban hospital serving a 75 percent Latino community recognized that one of the biggest health care problems among Latino males is diabetes. The hospital created a successful program that serves, and hence captures, that market. Also, by paying attention to community patterns, they found that the area churches were centers around which residents congregated. The hospital provided nurses, who worked like private practice public health nurses, once a week at each church. People in the community could thus come to the church to get their health care questions answered and find out where to go for help. Prenatal education in Spanish is given free, with attendance made even more enticing by prizes such as child car seats. In addition, the hospital has a Women, Infants, and Children (WIC) program on site. When women come for nutrition, counseling, and classes, they see the hospital, learn about other programs provided, and build trust in the institution. This increased comfort translates into business and revenue. The hospital has found a way to thrive economically by providing care to an underserved, lower socioeconomic community.

Another example of a hospital finding an opportunity in the changing demographic composition of its community is Methodist Hospital in Arcadia, California. This suburban area of Los Angeles is in the San Gabriel Valley, home of one of the largest Asian, especially Chinese, populations in the United States. In fact, according to Elaine Vandeventer, director of education at Methodist Hospital, 50 to 60 percent of the students in Arcadia's schools are Asian. Realizing that the hospital's patient base was increasingly Chinese and that greater tolerance and adaptability could be keys to survival in a competitive economy helped the institution to investigate this emerging market and seek to meet its needs. What the hospital found was that in addition to the long-term residents and the recently arrived families of Chinese businessmen, another significant group was using the hospital. Because of restrictive reproductive policies, many Chinese women were coming to the United States to have a second child, for which they self-paid.

To serve this specific market and meet the needs of the resident Asian community, the hospital made significant adaptations. First, Chinese translation services were added and translators were oriented to American medical practices. The Chinese interpreters are full-time employees who work out of the ER. In addition, a Chinese marketing professional was hired and Chinese options were added to meal menus. Cultural diversity guest relations training was given to staff and physicians to help them understand and be more effective with their diverse patients. Diabetes education for Chinese patients was added. Even electric incense burners were provided. The cumulative effect of these measures was both top-quality care and service.

The changing demographics of a health care organization's service area and workforce presents both challenges and opportunities. Finding ways to capitalize on the potential benefits and deal with the accompanying challenges is critical to quality care and financial survival.

2

The Dimensions of
Health Care Diversity

- A postsurgery patient in great discomfort asks for pain
  medication and is admonished by his foreign-born nurse
  not to act like a baby.
- An elderly patient complains and asks for a different
  physical therapist (PT), one who is older and has more
  experience, because she does not think the young
  PT working with her knows what she is doing.
- Staff in the ER of an inner-city hospital express frustration
  at the large family groups that crowd the waiting area when
  they accompany patients seeking emergency treatment.
- Female nurses on the med/surgery unit complain that some
  of the male physicians with whom they work treat them in a
  demeaning way, as handmaidens rather than as professional
  partners in caregiving.

As these situations show, diversity plays a role in health care,
in both patient-staff interactions and intrastaff relationships. In the
examples just presented, ethnicity, age, and gender played key roles.
These and other dimensions, such as income, geographic location,
and education, influence both staff and patient opportunities, expectations, and assumptions about others. They also influence
beliefs and attitudes about such health care issues as

- What is top-quality care?
- Who can be trusted to provide it?
- What is the patient's role in the process?
- What is the meaning of and proper response to pain, illness, and suffering?

Maya Angelou's eloquent poem "Human Family" concludes

I note the obvious differences between each sort and type,
but we are more alike my friend, than we are unalike.[1]

If this is so, it is understandable that so many people ask, "Why do we have to focus so much on the differences?" One seminar participant, Tabiri Chukunta, coordinator of diversity at St. Peters Medical Center in New Brunswick, New Jersey, responded aptly when he said, "It's not our similarities that have caused all our problems but rather our differences."[2]

The four layers of diversity illustrated in Figure 2.1—personality, internal dimensions, external dimensions, and organizational dimensions—and the many factors they contain, offer a framework for considering the role that differences among people play in health care settings, in employee interactions with patients and visitors as well as in communications among coworkers, physicians, and other staff.

Personality: The Unique Core

One physician says something and patients and staff laugh, while another can say the same thing and they bristle. Why do some patients rub staff the wrong way and some have the opposite effect? The answer may have to do with the most basic factor about human beings: personality. Each person, whether brought up in a village or city, illiterate or degreed, young or old, has a unique style of interacting with others that affects that person's effectiveness in

Figure 2.1 The Four Layers of Diversity.

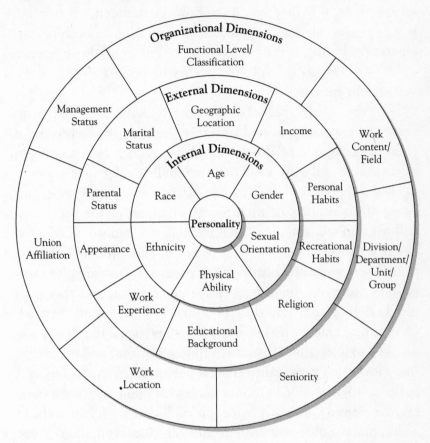

Source: Lee Gardenswartz and Anita Rowe, *Diverse Teams at Work* (Burr Ridge, Ill.: Irwin, 1994), p. 33. Internal dimensions and external dimensions adapted from Marilyn Loden and Judy Rosener, *Workforce America!* (Burr Ridge, Ill.: Irwin, 1991), pp. 18–19. Reprinted by permission of *The Western Journal of Medicine.*

communicating, influences others' reactions, and helps or hinders relationships. Whether a nurse, technician, therapist, or physician is seen as intimidating or approachable, irritating or soothing, fascinating or boring, curt or welcoming, can make all the difference in his or her ability to work effectively with colleagues or give the best care to patients.

To explore this aspect of diversity we sometimes ask staff members to pair up with a trusted coworker, preferably one who is from another background. Without speaking, each person writes ten words that describe his or her own personality and style of interacting with others. Words such as *approachable, analytical, intense, fun-loving, shy, nurturing,* or *organized* might appear on the list. Then, still without speaking, each staff member writes down words that describe the other person. They then compare their lists, sharing their descriptions and hearing their partner's. They are often surprised at some of the differences in perceptions, and they gain insight from hearing how these personality traits are demonstrated. One administrator who saw himself as approachable and soft was shocked to learn that his staff saw him as fearsome and intimidating. How one's personality style is perceived by coworkers and patients influences one's interactions with them. The same traits may be viewed differently by people of disparate backgrounds. In addition, some traits may be more difficult to deal with than others. In diverse settings there is a need for everyone involved to become more sensitive to the potential negative perceptions of one's own traits, as well as to work more effectively with the difficult aspects of others' personalities.

Internal Dimensions of Diversity: Powerful Influencers of Identity, Opportunity, and Expectations

Beyond the central core of personality, the six internal dimensions of diversity, referred to as primary dimensions by Marilyn Loden and Judy Rosener,[3] have a profound influence on how we see ourselves and others, on how others see us, and on what our expectations are for ourselves and those around us. What is more, these dimensions are for the most part out of our control. Gender, race, age, sexual orientation, ethnicity, and physical ability are generally standard equipment rather than options we choose. Let us take a look at how each of these dimensions might influence interactions between patients and staff and among employees.

Age

Assumptions about age may emerge when patients select among a twenty-something, forty-something, or sixty-something physician. They may also emerge in staff hiring decisions, or in practitioners' preferences in dealing with patients in these three generations. Knee-jerk assumptions about age, whether acknowledged or not, often underlie reactions.

Age does make a difference. The era in which one grows up puts an indelible imprint on one's values and expectations. Consider the differences, for example, between a postwar baby boomer raised by depression-era parents and a generation Xer growing up in the greater affluence of the 1980s. Maturity levels and life experiences leave their mark as well. Cultural factors may also influence a person's attitude toward age. For example, in Asia elders are generally respected for their wisdom, while in the United States age is often seen as a detriment to be concealed with antiwrinkle cosmetics, hair dye, and plastic surgery.

Among staff, assumptions abound at both ends of the spectrum. Younger physicians, nurses, and managers sometimes complain that they are not being taken seriously and that they are accused of wanting too much too soon. Some older nurses and business office staff feel that they are discounted because of their age and deemed to be averse to change and resistant to learning new procedures. What happens when young and old meet in the examining room, at the hiring interview, across the admissions desk, or at the bedside?

Gender

While it is no longer a shock to encounter a woman physician or a male nurse, expectations about gender roles still linger, if not in the forefront then in the deeper recesses of our consciousness. One of the authors remembers an incident when her mother was rushed to the ER with a heart problem. Having been told that the cardiologist, whom they had not met, would meet them there, the author was on the lookout for the specialist. As they were rushed in, she saw a woman with a clipboard and immediately assumed she was the intake clerk. When she noticed that this staff member had a stethoscope around her neck, she revised her assessment and mentally labeled the woman an ER nurse. Of course, you have already figured out that the mystery woman was the cardiologist. This author would vehemently defend the right of women to be physicians in any specialty. Yet as a result of society's socialization she had unconsciously fallen into the gender-role expectations that affect all of us. One hospital with a physician referral service reports that the most common request is for a female physician. It seems that callers to the service have some strong preconceived notions about male and female physicians and have attached more positive expectations to females.

Finally, men and women communicate differently. Staff at one HMO report that female physicians spend three to five minutes longer with patients per visit. Deborah Tannen, in her book *You Just Don't Understand*,[4] tells us that men communicate "vertically," as a means of establishing a hierarchy of order and power and to solve problems. Women, however, communicate "horizontally," interacting to form relationships and share feelings and reactions. This difference can lead to subtle barriers in transmitting information and to even more subtle assumptions. He may be seen as cold and insensitive, she may be perceived as wasting time.

The same behavior may be seen differently when exhibited by the two sexes. An aggressive male physician may be seen as in charge and a leader, while a female physician behaving in the same way might be viewed as pushy and arrogant. A female nurse asking for time off for a child's school play may be seen as not dedicated enough to her work, while her male colleague might be viewed as a model father for making the same request. Reactions to pain as well as complaints and symptoms are often treated differently depending on the gender of the patient because of differing gender role expectations.

Think about the attitudes and beliefs about gender differences in your health care setting. For example, some staff members may report feeling more comfortable in same-sex work groups or working with patients of the same gender; some may strongly prefer reporting to a manager of the opposite sex; and still others may find it awkward to be the only man or woman on a case team.

Gender makes a difference not only in the diseases to which one is susceptible but also in the amount of research dollars given to studying disease. Women have historically been on the short end of the research stick. Although women's health is now starting to get more attention, and more money is being provided for research into women's health issues, assumptions about, for example, the causes of heart disease are frequently based on male populations. Also, some important cultural norms are highly shaped by gender, which can have an impact on treatment and doctor-patient relationships. In the Asian Pacific, Middle East, or Mexico and Central America, for example, a high value is placed on privacy and propriety. This results in awkwardness for women who need to be examined by or to disrobe for male physicians. Once these physicians know this, they can make arrangements to have female nurse practitioners involved as much as possible to minimize patients' discomfort with male doctors. Among the most dynamic medical practice groups we have seen in Southern California are those that are feverishly trying to hire excellent female physicians. They tell us that women patients frequently request female physicians because seeing a woman doctor increases their comfort significantly at a time when they already feel anxious. Paying attention to the population you serve and doing some work ahead of time to match competent physicians of both genders with your patient base will be a smart move that serves everyone well.

Ethnicity

Another aspect of diversity is ethnicity. An individual's nationality or ethnic background includes such aspects as native language and culture. Some people proudly proclaim their heritage and define themselves as Mexican American, Arab American, or Polish American. Others label themselves only by their country of origin, for example, calling themselves Cuban, Russian, or South African. Some with multiple or unknown nationalities in their background identify themselves as just plain American.

These ethnic differences can bring variations in cultural norms, holiday observances, food preferences, language proficiency, and group affiliation. Cultural influences can also direct a person's health care beliefs and preferences, from folk medicine, healers, and holistic or natural remedies to high-tech procedures and complex tests. Culture can influence a person's beliefs about illness. In some cases illness is seen as a punishment from God, while in others it could be seen as the neglect or abuse of one's body. Some cultures perceive sickness as resulting from a random invasion by bacteria or viruses, while others view it as the result of a spiritual imbalance.

Ethnicity may also correlate to patients' beliefs about disease and their response to treatment. For example, Latinos express greater fear of breast, uterine, and lung cancer, go less often to physicians for screening, and show more pessimism about successful outcomes. They also exhibit a greater lack of personal power or control in reducing cancer risk than do other groups.[5] Finally, a number of health problems with genetic components are more prevalent in certain groups. Examples of these are Tay-Sachs among Jews, sickle cell anemia among African Americans, lactose intolerance among Asians and Asian-Americans, and diabetes among Native Americans.[6]

One's native language and proficiency in an adopted one are also aspects of ethnicity. Fluency in English is often seen as a requisite for competency as a health care provider in the United States, and as a bonus when being treated as a patient. In focus groups we are often told by non-native English speakers that they feel that staff and patients assume they are less intelligent and able because of their accented English. Conversely, monolingual English-speaking staff often find themselves at a disadvantage; they experience frustration when they cannot understand patients or other staff because of a language barrier or when groups of coworkers speak another language in front of them.

An often more subtle manifestation of ethnicity can be seen in culture, the behavioral software that guides behavior. Not making eye contact is seen by some cultures as deceitful or unassertive, while other cultures see it as a sign of respect shown to elders and authority figures. Some people who are ill may want a private room and only immediate family visiting, while others might need the constant company of an extended family group to aid in recovery. Some nurses expect to be involved in decision making on their teams and enjoy actively participating in brainstorming and discussions at meetings. Others, however, might expect the manager to give direction and would feel more comfortable giving careful, private forethought to ideas before presenting them.

Individuals are generally unaware of these subtle cultural influences and assume that their preferences are universal. What is more, one's own rules are generally regarded as right or as better than those of others. The coworker who stands closer than we are comfortable with is seen as pushy; the one who stands too far away is seen as aloof. The patient who nods and says yes even though she does not understand is seen not as respectful and desiring harmony but as unassertive or not truthful, while the one who asks too many questions and disagrees is seen as difficult or uncooperative.

As you consider the interplay of the different ethnicities in your facility, consider those cultural differences that cause obstacles. The more health care providers know about the different ethnic backgrounds of their patients and coworkers, as well as the influences of their own ethnic backgrounds, the more effective they will be in meeting and providing effective care. (The influence of culture is discussed in much greater depth and specificity in Chapters Three and Four.)

Physical Ability

It is estimated that about 43 million Americans have some kind of physical disability.[7] Some of these impairments are obvious, such as paralysis or blindness. Others, including hearing loss or dyslexia, are not so readily apparent. People with such disabilities will be among your patients and your colleagues. Those who have physical disabilities often comment on the discomfort they perceive able-bodied individuals to have in dealing with them. They report being ignored frequently in a group or having questions about them directed at a friend, partner, or attendant, as though they were not present. It might be helpful to ask patients with special needs to help you understand the best way to treat them. They undoubtedly know more about their capabilities than you do. In the same way, staff members with physical limitations may have creative suggestions about how they could accomplish tasks that you might have assumed were out of their ability range. Installing TDD lines for those with hearing impairments, having signs and elevator buttons in Braille, and providing sign language interpreters at meetings and public education sessions are adaptations many hospitals have made to meet the needs of staff and patients with disabilities.

Sexual Orientation

Human sexual orientation can be viewed as a continuum, with some individuals being heterosexual, some bisexual, and some gay or lesbian. Patients and colleagues will fall along all points of the spectrum. While those who are heterosexual generally express their

orientation inadvertently and in casual conversations when referring to wives, husbands, and family activities, those who are gay,
lesbian, or bisexual generally do not have such freedom. Some
openly discuss their sexual orientation and others do not. The
range of reactions by employees to colleagues' disclosure of being
gay or lesbian is equally wide. In some health care settings, jokes
and innuendoes about homosexuality still cause snickers and raised
eyebrows, while in others same-sex partner benefits have been
accepted for a while.

Consider the assumptions and expectations about sexual orientation that exist in your hospital. Are physicians engaged in AIDS
research assumed to be gay? Are lesbian and gay patients reticent to
disclose their sexual orientation because they fear they will get
poorer treatment? Do heterosexual staff imagine that homosexual
coworkers of the same gender will make passes at them? One staff
member explained that in discussions of birth control all women are
incorrectly assumed to be heterosexual. Often the interview goes
like this: "Are you sexually active?" "Well, yeah." "Well then, you
should be on birth control."

Race

Many individuals proudly claim to be "color blind," often mistak-
enly assuming that this is a compliment to a person of color.
According to Janet Elsea, in her book *The Four Minute Sell*, in the
United States skin color is the first thing we notice about one
another.[8] According to her research, gender and age are second
and third. Statistics from many aspects of American life tell us that
race makes a difference in treatment in all walks of life. For example, a 1992 study by the Federal Reserve Bank of Boston reports
that "mortgage applications of non-whites were rejected 60 percent
more often than for whites with the same level of income and credit
history."[9] Such inequities in treatment are also seen in health care.
Jill Klessig reports that racism is still a problem in the medical establishment; less intense care is given to African American patients

and they tend to be more stereotyped than others.[10] And according to an article in *Occupational Medicine*, the mortality rate for African American males is 50 percent higher than the rate for white males and females, with the life expectancy of African American males and females being seven and five years less, respectively, than for whites.[11]

The dimension of race also plays a role in physical vulnerabilities. For example, cardiovascular disease is more prevalent among African Americans; it is the leading cause of death among African American males. Eighty-five percent of African American women forty-five to sixty-five years old have hypertension, and younger women (twenty-five to forty-four) have a 2.6 times greater rate of hypertension than white women in the same age group. Diabetes is another health problem more prevalent among African Americans, with females having a 50 percent higher rate than their white counterparts. It is also more prevalent among Mexican Americans, who have a two to three times greater risk than whites of having the disease.[12]

External Dimensions

Beyond internal dimensions there are many factors relating to our life experiences and choices that influence our opportunities, attitudes, and situations, as well as the assumptions that others have about us.

Religion

Once considered a Judeo-Christian country, the United States is increasingly becoming home to people of a much wider array of religions. Mosques as well as Hindu and Buddhist temples are no longer rarities in cities across the country. Not only does religion give many people a basic set of values and rules that guides their lives, such as the Ten Commandments or the Noble Eightfold Path, but it also prescribes observances, rituals, and holidays. Seventh Day Adventists and Observant Jews who consider Saturday the Sabbath would not want to work on that day. A Muslim employee who prays five times a day would not be available for noon staff meetings. Non-Christian patients and their families might not feel at home in a chapel or meditation room adorned with crucifixes or other sectarian symbols. A Jehovah's Witness employee might object to a birthday party in her honor because her religion forbids such celebrations.

The religious beliefs of patients may also necessitate certain practices, such as a priest's visit and communion for an ill Catholic or Eastern Orthodox patient, and Extreme Unction, commonly known as last rights, for the dying. For others, special procedures upon death before the patient is removed from the hospital room, such as turning the body to face a certain direction or the lighting of candles, may be required. Finally, food preferences may be directed by religious rules—Kosher for Jews, Halal for Muslims, and a vegetarian diet for Seventh Day Adventists.

Education

An individual's type and level of education are clearly factors in the professional world, where credentials and résumés are required. Degrees are often noted on organizational name tags, and the type of training one has—medical, business, or scientific—as well as one's level of education—high school diploma, MBA, Ph.D., or M.D.—influences credibility and opportunities. Educational experience may also have an impact on a patient's attitude toward health care and caregivers. For less-educated patients, the hospital or clinic may feel literally like a foreign country. In such a setting, they may feel intimidated or be less articulate in putting forth questions and getting procedures clarified. They may also feel less entitled to ask questions, or find it difficult to indicate a lack of understanding when interacting with someone with more education.

Marital Status

Married, single, divorced, widowed—you might ask, what difference does it make? To a Southeast Asian obstetrics patient, being asked if she was married was a terrible insult, impugning her respectableness and insulting her husband.[13] To a seminar participant in one of our training sessions, marital status was a major determinant in selecting personnel. "I never hire anyone who is single," she proclaimed, relating a list of assumptions she had made about single peoples' supposed lack of responsibility, commitment, work ethic, and dependability. Though her stereotyping has illegal consequences and is extreme, marital status connotes different things to different people. And it does not have the same meaning for male and female employees, with married men sometimes assumed to be more stable and settled, and married women in their childbearing years seen as more of a dependability risk. Marital status can also have an impact on work group relationships. Single people often complain about being expected to do overtime, extra shifts, and weekend work, while those with children in day care find it disruptive to get to early morning meetings, deal with last-minute shift changes, or be called on or off duty with little warning.

In addition, marital status norms vary by ethnic group and may affect the socioeconomic status of patients. For example, 44 percent of Puerto Rican households and 43 percent of African American households are headed by single females, compared to 13 percent of white households.[14]

Income

Staff income levels often affect esteem, job satisfaction, and stress levels. For patients, the amount one earns can determine access to health care as well as the level of care received. According to a Kaiser Permanente report, 40 to 50 percent of Latinos are uninsured, generally because of their concentration in lower-income jobs with few or no health care benefits.[15] Income can also provide or limit access to education, transportation, and nutrition. An elderly patient on a fixed income may have a difficult time getting transportation to medical appointments. A young single mother just getting by with the help of government assistance may be able to get care only at a distant clinic where she must wait long hours to be treated. A "working poor" patient without prescription benefits may not be able to afford expensive medications.

Parental Status

Having children means additional responsibility for both staff and patients. Child-care arrangements and last-minute emergencies due to children's illnesses can sometimes interfere with appointments and scheduled responsibilities. In one urban hospital, a staff nurse on night shift was repeatedly admonished for making personal calls while on the job. When she did not stop the prohibited behavior, the nursing administrator sat down and had a heart-to-heart talk with her. After learning that continued infractions would cost her her job, the nurse finally confessed that she was a single parent with three young children and had no child care. She had been calling home to make sure her children were all right. Once the truth came to light, the administrator helped her arrange affordable and appropriate child care so the nurse could focus on her job, secure in the knowledge that her children were safe.

In many hospital and clinic waiting areas, a children's play area equipped with toys and books keeps young ones occupied while their sometimes stressed and anxious parents wait. Finally, in many hospitals children are allowed to visit patients on designated floors.

Appearance

Although many of us have been taught not to judge a book by its cover, appearance does influence our opinions about others as well as our own self-esteem. One seminar participant, in lovely African garb of Kente cloth, related that she was advised that her choice of clothing put distance between her and some of those she served. It seemed that they viewed her ethnic dress as a sign of black militancy and as an adversarial stance toward whites. Another seminar participant, a brewery worker, had been struck by a heart attack while on the job and was rushed to the local hospital by ambulance. He was shocked and insulted when he was asked by three health care workers if he was on cocaine. Undoubtedly his long hair and his thirty-something youthful look led them to make an inaccurate assumption about the cause of his medical problem.

Dress can also have an impact on interstaff relationships. One wise boss recognized that gender differences were causing conflicts on his staff. The traditionally male workforce in one department was having a difficult time accepting female employees. The manager put everyone in gender-neutral jumpsuit uniforms that helped staff identify with their profession. Employees were then able to look beyond gender differences and see one another not as men or women but as skilled professionals.

What are staff members' reactions to patients or other staff with pierced noses, lips, or tongues? How about your attitude toward those with tattoos? Shaved heads? Men with turbans or yarmulkes? Women wearing head scarves or facial veils? Staff in lab coats, uniforms, or civilian dress? Which are appearance turnoffs for you or others? Consider how these reactions might hinder service.

Personal Habits

Personal habits such as smoking, drinking, or exercising can influence health. They can also be catalysts for building or hindering collegial relationships. Staff who aerobicize or go on lunchtime walks, take smoking breaks, or go out together for beers after work may form bonds that may strengthen work relationships. They may also exclude other staff members who do not share the same habits. These activities can also enhance or hinder one's health. In addition, substance abuse problems affect not only health and performance but safety as well. In one suburban hospital, a patient behaving irrationally because of the influence of a hallucinogenic drug injured himself and scared staff when he jumped from the window of his room to the parking lot floors below.

Recreational Habits

Gardening? Soccer? Needlework? Fishing? Basketball? Recreational preferences form another part of the diversity mosaic. Camaraderie builds among those who share a common activity. Talking sports with a young fan may be the quickest way to build rapport with an adolescent patient. Networking and relationship building for staff may take place on the golf course or by watching the Super Bowl. Some activities serve as levelers, bringing together people from many walks of life and levels in the organization. Other activities can exclude people, such as immigrants who may live for soccer not football, or coworkers who do not care about sports at all. Recreational activities can bring people together or keep them apart in your organization. Some activities, such as soccer or ten-kilometer runs, can help build relationships within the diverse community served.

Geographic Location

The areas where staff members and patients were raised and in which they presently live have a bearing on behaviors, attitudes, and access. Cultural norms and paces differ in big cities and small towns, rural areas and suburbs, parts of the United States and regions of the world. The neighborhoods where patients live may or may not be safe. Where a facility is located may be more or less convenient to patients and more or less welcoming to different groups. It is also important to remember that welcome lies in the eye of the beholder. When two hospitals from different parts of one city merged, staff assumed that patients from the poorer, other-side-of-the-tracks community, who had been served by the older of the two hospitals, would welcome coming to the other hospital, in a more affluent, touted-as-better part of town. They were surprised to find that this was not the case. The diverse patients from the older facility were not at all sure that they would be welcomed nor well treated by the mostly white staff at the newer hospital.

Place of origin can be particularly significant for refugees. Diseases such as malaria, tuberculosis, hepatitis B, and malnutrition are often much more prevalent among recently arrived refugees. Chronic medical problems such as posttraumatic stress disorder, depression, and anxiety are seen among refugees who have resided in the United States for a longer period.[16]

Work Experience

Computer whizzes and technophobes, typists and technicians, therapists and nurses, accountants and transporters, physicians and housekeepers—all come together and make contributions in your organization. Yet often some experiences are valued over others. Are specialists held above generalists? Differences can bring value to teams when the contributions of each member are utilized. Teams can also shut people out by discounting their experience.

Certain types of work may be associated with particular ethnic and racial groups, who may experience higher rates of health risks. For example, Latinos, because of their overrepresentation in farming, manufacturing, and construction, have nearly twice the rate of disability from work-related injury as nonminority workers.[17] Work experience may also trigger assumptions about patients. Staff may subtly react differently to taking care of a professor, a day laborer, a physician, a truck driver, a lawyer, or a welfare recipient.

Organizational Dimensions

Beyond the internal and external influences on an individual are organizational categories, which can be the source of assumptions and opportunities, helping or hindering staff teamwork and employee effectiveness.

Functional Level or Classification

No matter how flattened the management structure, all organizations have some kind of hierarchy, a pecking order that delineates the chain of command. Though the definition of reporting relationships may be the purpose of such a chain, it has other outcomes, both creating a sense of order and security and, at the same time, causing barriers because of an often-perceived caste system. Levels or classification labels may serve as coveted signs of status, indications of pay differentials, or implied sources of power.

Levels and titles also affect esteem. One supervisor was left with no staff when her department was downsized. This Chinese-born staff member went to her boss, herself an immigrant from the Philippines, to plead that her title not be taken away. She explained that she would lose face in her community if she lost the title of supervisor. The boss, caring more about having a satisfied, productive employee than a logical organization chart, responded affirmatively.

Often rubs about these differences in level emerge in strange ways. In one organization a hot topic for parking lot conversations was water. It seems that bottled water was found only on the executive floor, with all other floors having water fountains. Clearly the issue was one of power, esteem, and status, with water being the symbol. At an HMO, an employee association made up of staff from all levels of the organization who belonged to an ethnic support group found this dimension to have an impact. Hourly employees, whose input and involvement were needed by the group, were unable to attend meetings scheduled at lunch or in early morning hours. Because of hourly staff's thirty-minute lunchtimes and inflexible work hours, the association began to be composed of mostly salaried employees, who had more leeway in their schedules. This factor also had an impact on attendance at résumé-writing and job-finding workshops held by the association. Hourly staff who were in danger of being laid off and who could benefit most from the sessions were unable to attend.

Management Status

It is rare to find an organization, whether in or out of health care, in which there is not an "us versus them" feeling between nonmanagerial and managerial staff. We are frequently pulled to the side and told by staff in training sessions that they would be more candid if managers were not in the group. Although the fear is often greater than the reality, and the barrier does not break down if groups remain separated, the rift is a common one. People recently promoted into their first supervisory position frequently report that the transition to management is gut wrenching, and that relationships with former peers are irrevocably altered. In fact, in one hospital the participant notebook for new supervisor training opens with the following statement: "Welcome to management. Your life will never be the same."

Because of differences in responsibilities and perspectives, the concerns and viewpoints of managerial and nonmanagerial personnel are often not the same. These differences can be a benefit, helping a staff or department to get a fuller picture of an issue in order to solve a problem. However, they can sometimes put people at odds with one another and trigger assumptions and stereotypes. Comments such as "They don't care about us and they don't want to hear about our pressures" are heard from one side of the divide. "They just want to punch in and punch out; they don't care about the bigger picture" is a complaint voiced from the other camp.

Department/Unit/Work Group

The professional home for employees is not the organization as a whole but usually their own department or unit. It is here that relationships are built and careers are developed. Yet all departments are not created equal. It is common for there to be images and stereotypes about specific departments or units. Reputations precede the people from these departments. Staff in some departments are well respected as high performing, while those from other departments are seen as troublemakers. Think about what people say about various departments in your hospital. The reputation of units, shifts, and groups in your organization will influence others' reactions to them as well as the morale of the staff themselves.

These assumptions often play out in what is a frequently voiced problem in health care: obstacles to interdepartmental communication and cooperation. Cross-functional teams that bring people from different parts of the hospital or clinic together to solve problems or delineate procedures often help break down some of these walls.

Union Affiliation

Whether employees are union members or not and the kind of relationships that exist between union and nonunion employees can add another wrinkle to the diversity fabric of staff. Union membership on the part of patients can indicate strong health care benefits as well.

Work Location

Whether one works in the main building or in a trailer in the parking lot, at a remote clinic, or in the ER can make a difference in staff members' viewpoints and attitudes as well as in others' perceptions about them. Not only does work location influence communication, but it can also be seen as a sign of importance or value. Consider the image of the various work locations in your hospital, especially those that are favored or ignored.

Seniority

A revered tradition in organizations is the value placed on seniority. Promotions, schedules, vacations, overtime, and other perks are often doled out on this basis. Generally the hierarchy of seniority is more valued by mature employees who have been socialized in a system where longevity was a sign of loyalty and commitment, and by those from hierarchical cultures who see age as commanding respect and bringing wisdom. Union contracts and organizational policies have traditionally used seniority as a fair and accepted way to give advantages. While job security and loyalty of long-term employees are often touted as the upsides of seniority, there may be disadvantages as well. During downsizings, complaints are occasionally heard that some of the best employees are let go because of their short time with the organization while those with more seniority are kept regardless of competence.

Work Content/Field

The kind of work that people do makes for still another difference. Social workers and accountants probably do not see things in the same way. Neither do lawyers and nurses or physicians and human resource staff. Each type of work is a subculture of its own that gives its members a methodology for defining and working out problems. In one biotechnical firm a manager revealed that her most difficult diversity barrier was not one of gender, age, or culture but of work content. As a human resource professional, she faced her biggest challenge in communicating with engineers. "We talk different languages," she said.

In addition, each kind of work has its own status. Jokes abound about mothers wanting their daughters to marry doctors, not plumbers or ditch diggers. What fields of work are held in highest regard in your hospital? Are researchers more esteemed than clinicians? Are physicians considered more valuable than marketing professionals?

Analyzing the Impact of Diversity Dimensions in Your Organization

How can you deal with all these differences, both on staff and among patients? The place to start is to analyze which differences are the most significant and what impact they have. You might find it helpful to think first of your hospital or clinic as a whole, asking yourself which of these dimensions is the most significant in interactions with patients and among staff. As you consider the dimensions, focus on the specific consequences in care of patients and in teamwork among staff.

It is even more helpful to discuss your perceptions with a group of coworkers. Which dimensions make the most difference in how staff and patients are treated, and how are differences shown? What are the consequences for your institution in terms of teamwork? Delivery of quality care? Cost effectiveness? Which are areas of inequity that create obstacles to care? These discussions can help you identify opportunities to be taken advantage of as well as problems to be solved.

Analyzing the Impact of Your Own Diversity Dimensions on You as a Health Care Professional

As a health care professional, you are one of the primary tools of your trade. Your diversity factors and how they play out in your interactions with coworkers, patients, physicians, and visitors significantly influence your relationships and your effectiveness.

Consider each of the diversity dimensions and its impact on you and select a few that have been the most important in forming the person you are now. Think about the most important values, rules, or lessons you have learned from each dimension, then about the effect this aspect of diversity has had on your professional life and your work. For example, if, as a woman, gender has been a primary influence, you might have been brought up to be nonassertive, accepting, and nurturing, and you might have been taught that you should always be ladylike. The impact may be that you are great at maintaining positive relationships with coworkers and building rapport with patients. However, you may also find it difficult to confront physicians or deal with demanding family members.

If because of your generation or culture you were raised to work hard, be prompt, and not make excuses, you may be thorough, responsible, and hardworking. Conversely, you may find yourself getting irritated with others who do not share your values about time or your work ethic.

Analyzing Your Own Attitudes Toward Differences

Providing health care is an intensely personal process in which you are asked to interact with others on a more intimate level than is required in the business world. Making a human-to-human connection is critical to developing the rapport necessary for optimal care. You are an essential element in making that connection. As a human being you have your own reactions to, attitudes about, and preferences for various diversity dimensions. You may feel more comfortable with some groups than with others, find some practices offensive, or see some behaviors as irritating. You are entitled to your own feelings and perceptions. We all have them. But to be effective as a health care provider in a diverse environment, you need to be aware of your feelings and perceptions, and you need to make active choices about your behavior based on a clear recognition of them. If left unacknowledged, these attitudes and perceptions may sabotage the most clinically correct care or the most brilliant plan, hindering your ability to be successful.

Doing some introspection is helpful. Consider your attitudes about differences and in which dimensions you find the greatest discomfort. Also think about how these reactions influence your interactions with coworkers or patients in a particular group. Finally, spend time thinking about what you can do to increase your feeling of ease in such situations. The following chapters can help you understand some of these differences, as well as your own reactions to them.

As you can see, the impact of the many diversity dimensions is multifaceted and makes for complex interplays when patients, families, staff, and physicians interact. A good starting point in dealing with this complexity is to begin by discussing with coworkers the varied perceptions you may have about the effect these differences have on caregiving and teamwork. From there you can begin to identify issues and obstacles that hinder care and cooperation, as well as the opportunities that exist in such a rich mix.

3

The Truth About Cultural Programming

"Physiology is physiology." "We've all got the same basic equipment." You may have heard such sentiments expressed when the issue of cultural differences is brought up. These comments may be accurate, but they express only part of the truth. While we do share similar "hardware" with others of our species, we differ in our "software," the cultural rules and values that program our behavior. Without this cultural programming we would be as nonfunctional as a computer without software.

Culture guides our everyday behavior and tells us how to interpret others' actions. It helps us deal with life's problems and interact socially, showing us what to do in a variety of situations, from when to make eye contact and how close to stand, to the way to address someone or how to discipline a child. It also directs how we express pain, react to illness, and view suffering. No society could function without such commonly accepted behavioral norms. The difficulty in a multicultural environment is that there may be many different, and sometimes confusing and even incompatible, software programs operating. In such settings the risk of miscommunication and conflict is higher and the ability to build rapport and trusting relationships is more difficult than in homogenous cultures.

Realities of Cultural Programming

What makes things even more complex are the following realities about culture and how it operates:

- Culture is not overt.
- We are all essentially ethnocentric.
- We observe, interpret, then act.
- We may not know when we are offending others.
- Awareness and knowledge increase our choices.
- Understanding one's own software is a first step.

Culture is not overt. Culture is powerful, yet subtle. Cultural rules are usually not discussed unless a rule is broken. Then the transgressor may be admonished for having bad manners, for being poorly raised, or for not considering others. We operate with the rules of our cultural software on automatic pilot, unaware of their influence on our actions. Like a fish who does not know it is in water until it is taken out, we define our cultural rules only when we encounter different ones that cause us to make comparisons. It is generally only when we meet people operating with a different set of assumptions and values that we become aware of our own.

We are all essentially ethnocentric. Because our cultural software is so much a part of us and because it is shared, we rarely question it and we naturally assume our rules, values, and beliefs to be correct. We see behaviors from our own perspective and tend to judge negatively those who have different software. The person who speaks too loudly is labeled aggressive, the one who arrives late is considered rude, the one who claims a friend as a relative is seen as deceitful. Staff in one pediatric clinic serving a working class immigrant community saw their ethnocentrism twice. Originally dealing with a mainly Latino population, they frequently complained about these clients being so passive. When the demographics of the area changed with the arrival of new immigrants from Armenia, the complaints changed. Staff began commenting on how aggressive these newcomers were. The software of both groups differed from that of the staff, and both were judged using the staff's own preferences as the norm.

Ethnocentrism, using one's own cultural rules as the basis of comparison, is a normal human phenomenon. It is only when we recognize that our rules are not universal that we begin to question our reactions, expand our understanding, and enable ourselves to build relationships with people of other cultures.

We observe, interpret, then act. When we encounter another person's behavior we do not just observe what they are doing; we also attach meaning to the behavior and then act based on that meaning. Our interpretation about others' behaviors is based on our own software. For example, in Japan, one is often bumped by strangers on the street or in the subway. When no "excuse me" accompanies the offense, cultural programming may cause an American to react to what is felt to be rude and inconsiderate treatment. This is not the interpretation made by the Japanese, however, who do not consider bumping someone in public offensive at all and who would not expect an apology. Acting on the initial interpretation would be inappropriate in that context.

Knowledge gives us the ability to alter our interpretations. One manager, an American-born-and-bred male who supervised many Taiwanese staff members, was perplexed by one of their reactions. He complained that these employees were always "snickering" at him because they smiled and laughed when he explained procedures or gave directions to them. When he learned that for many Asians smiling and laughter is a sign of embarrassment and confusion, he quickly changed his interpretation of their behavior. Armed with this small bit of new knowledge, he understood them better and could find ways to work through whatever difficulties existed. Continuing to make incorrect assumptions about their behavior would have undoubtedly caused misunderstandings to escalate.

We may not know when we are offending others. Because we operate on the basis of our own set of meanings and assumptions, we may inadvertently offend others. Unknowingly we may hurt, demean, or show disrespect. One staff member helping an immigrant client fill out forms thought he was being sensitive. Knowing that this newcomer was not fluent in English and that the necessary paperwork was complex and confusing, he tried to put the client at ease. In attempting to create a relaxed atmosphere, he took his jacket off, smiled frequently, and engaged in joking banter with passing coworkers. The forms were completed and all seemed to go well, so he was surprised when the client called from home to complain about how rudely and disrespectfully he had been treated. It seems that in his culture respect would have been shown by a more formal demeanor and serious tone.

Awareness and knowledge increase our choices. According to organization development author and consultant John E. Jones, "Awareness precedes choice."[1] The authors would amend that statement to include knowledge as well as awareness. When we are no longer oblivious to what has previously directed our behavior, we can make conscious and perhaps more appropriate choices about our actions and reactions.

Understanding one's own software is a first step. Before you examine other cultural norms, it is helpful to get a deeper and clearer understanding of your own software program. Each individual's unique set of values, rules, and preferences is a product of many influences in the person's development, with parents, schools, neighborhoods, religious institutions, extended family, and friends often topping the list of cultural software shapers.

Take a few minutes to think about the major sources of your own software. For each of the sources, consider the values, rules, teachings, and lessons you learned, as well as their impact on your life and work. For example, your family may have instilled in you values of loyalty to family members, respect for elders, and duty toward one's parents. This may mean that you feel a tremendous obligation to care for your aging parents or to help out an ill sibling.

It may also mean that you find yourself irritated with patients' family members who do not show the concern for loved ones that you deem proper. Or you may be willing to cover for a coworker who needs to take an ill parent to a medical appointment.

You may have been raised to work hard, shoulder your responsibilities, and pay your own way in life. Does that make you resentful of patients on public assistance or coworkers who cut corners and just slide by? Or you may have been taught that the squeaky wheel gets the grease. Does that make you the spokesperson for every problem and issue on staff? It also may make you irritated with patients who smile, nod, and do not tell you much about their condition.

Dimensions of Culture That Influence Behavior

From how to talk with one's manager or what to eat for breakfast to the appropriate roles for men, women, and children or the meaning of a smile, culture encompasses the rules for interacting, solving problems, and making decisions. The following ten aspects of culture, proposed by Harris and Moran,[2] give us one way to categorize the universal experience of culture while exploring the range of differences within each aspect.

Sense of Self and Space

How close we stand to others, how or whether we touch, the level of formality we prefer, and the degree of openness we show are all parts of how we manage our sense of self and our physical space. "Too close for comfort" and "Get out of my space" are expressions of the need for some physical distance. Conversely, Edward Hall, the father of intercultural communication, tells us in his book *The Hidden Dimension*, in the Middle East people stand close enough to one another to feel each other's breath on their faces.[3] For those who prefer an arm's length between themselves and another individual, standing any closer may feel like an invasion or aggression. The person who expects a shorter distance may feel rebuffed by the one who continues to step away. Being crowded, jostled, and touched may feel like normal contact to some, while others find it unnerving and rude.

Even a handshake is culturally influenced. What is your assumption about a soft handshake? Do *weak*, *unassertive*, or *indecisive* come to mind? Yet in many parts of the world such a handshake is preferred over a bone-crunching, hearty grasp. In Asia, for example, a soft handshake with the left hand brought up under the clasped right hands is generally used as a sign of warmth and friendship.

Another difference between cultures relates to the level of formality that is preferred. In some cultures, introductions are made with both first and last names, and titles—such as Mr., Dr., Mrs., or Professor—are used to address each person being introduced. Health care staff may be addressed by position, such as Miss Nurse. People are expected to stand erectly, with no slouching or leaning allowed. To make explicit the level of formality required, many languages of the world use two forms of the word *you*, one familiar, the other formal, as in *Tu* and *Usted* in Spanish.

Finally, there is a range among cultures with regard to what may be discussed publicly and what must be kept private. Sharing one's ideas and thoughts at a meeting or brainstorming in a work team might be second nature to some people, but for someone reared in a culture such as that of Korea or Japan, offhand comments and "shooting from the hip" are not valued. Because words cannot be taken back, in these cultures careful thought is given before ideas are spoken aloud—and cultural admonitions caution that the wisest counsel is one's own.

In addition, speaking about personal problems, feelings, or intimate aspects of one's life, especially outside of the family, is discouraged in some cultures. In others it is considered healthy to open up and get things off your chest. One agency aimed at stopping domestic violence and sexual abuse found this cultural difference to be an obstacle in reaching out to its increasing number of Latino and Asian community members. Having bilingual hot-line counselors was not enough. Although women of many backgrounds who are survivors of abuse and assault often do not call the hot line to get help because of their sense of shame at divulging family secrets, the cultural programming for Latino and Asian women even more strongly discouraged their calling for help. Finding culturally appropriate ways to help these women has been a challenge that the organization continues to work on.

Suggestions Regarding Sense of Self and Space

- Start with a formal tone. You can always move to more casual interaction.

- Introduce yourself by full name and title or position.

- Address the other person by first and last name and title— Mr., Mrs., Miss, and so forth.

- Take your cue from the patient regarding handshakes, touch, and distance.

Communication and Language

"If only they would speak English, everything would be fine" is a common myth expressed in multicultural health care settings. For each of us the ability to communicate is a primary means of controlling our worlds. When that control is blocked, we often become frustrated. Yet communication goes far beyond language. Even in monolingual English-speaking environments, it is estimated that 50 to 90 percent of communication is nonverbal. Much is expressed by tone, gestures, and facial expressions. Rolled eyes, a sarcastic smirk, a welcoming smile, or raised eyebrows speak volumes. Yet, as with so much of our behavior, the rules about what certain gestures and looks mean are different from group to group. The OK sign made with the thumb and first finger is an obscene gesture in some parts of South America and the Mediterranean. A smile, seen by some as a sign of friendliness and welcome, may indicate stupidity and foolishness to a Korean, or a sexual come-on if from a woman to a man from the Middle East.

Eye contact is another human behavior that conveys different meanings depending on the group. "Look at me when I'm talking to you," many of us were told by a reprimanding parent. You may see direct eye contact as showing attentiveness and truthfulness. For most Asians, Native Americans, and some others, however, dropping one's eyes is a sign of respect and an expected behavior when in the presence of an authority figure or older person.

Finally, an even more subtle aspect of communication is the degree of directness. "Get to the point" and "Don't beat around the bush" are common expressions of the direct style common in the United States and other English-speaking countries. These cultures are seen as *low context*, with the meaning specifically expressed in the words. Great value is placed on exactness. The opposite of this orientation is that of Japan or Arabic-speaking cultures, which are seen as *high context*. In these cultures, meaning is found only partly in the words, with nonverbal cues, social relationships, and position contributing to the message as well. In high-context cultures, the listener is left to gather the clues and infer meaning in a much less direct way than in low-context cultures. What is not said may be as important as what is said.

This difference between direct/explicit and indirect/implicit styles can be seen in one of the most common sources of frustration, the yes-equals-no dilemma. For someone from an indirect, high-context culture, saying no directly may be considered rude and cause loss of face. A yes response may mean "Yes, I hear you," not "I agree" or "I understand." It may translate as "If I could explain it, I'd tell you that if you understood my position, could read my body language, and picked up on the tone of my voice you would know that my answer is really no. The problem is that my method of delivery is not direct and your low-context culture has taught you to pay attention only to my words."

Suggestions Regarding Communication

- Do not assume that a nod or a yes indicates understanding. Check for other signs of comprehension, such as performing a task or behaving according to directions.

- Avoid yes or no questions. Give choices instead.

- Consider that smiles and laughter may indicate confusion or embarrassment. Investigate to find the cause.

- Practice patience when interacting with someone who is less direct. See what you can learn from a different approach.

Dress and Appearance

- A pregnant Latina who uses public transportation to get to your clinic comes in wearing a silky dress and high heels.

- A young African American woman applying for a clerical job comes to the interview in a skin-tight, leopard-print jumpsuit.

Can you tell what's going on in each of these situations? How would you explain the dress and appearance of each of these women and how would you react to them?

Culture tells us how to dress and what is proper in different situations. Elizabeth Ortiz Valdez, CEO of the Concilio de Salud in Phoenix, sheds some light on how culture influenced the first situation described in the list. For the Latina, going to see the doctor is an important occasion and dressing up is a way to show her recognition of its importance and her respect for the health care provider. Ortiz Valdez suggests that rather than criticize the patient for wearing high heels while pregnant, the health care provider should compliment her on her appearance, then suggest low-heel shoes for walking.

In the second example, the interviewer found out that the

young woman had been told by everyone in her neighborhood that she was "lookin' good" in her jumpsuit. The job seeker wanted to put her best foot forward by wearing her most flattering outfit. The interviewer, who was aware enough to get beyond her initial assumptions based on dress, found that the applicant had the skills needed for the job. After the woman was hired, the interviewer spent time coaching her on appropriate attire for the workplace. Dress may make a social or political statement, it may be a form of artistic self-expression or a sign of wealth and prestige, or it may be just a necessity of life.

In addition to dress and grooming, hair and personal hygiene are also influenced by our cultural software. For example, religions and cultural rules may prescribe the covering of one's hair and body with head scarves, veils, or turbans. Body odor and the use of deodorants and perfumes are another area of cultural variation. One Peace Corps volunteer, a U.S.–born woman, related a fascinating incident. She was paired with a woman from another country to share a tent during their training. Having brought an abundant supply of grooming products—soap, toothpaste, shampoo, and deodorant—the American woman was well equipped. A few days later she was quite surprised when her tentmate remarked, "You don't smell like you're alive." Odor is in the nose of the beholder.

Suggestions Regarding Dress and Appearance

- Do not assume that body odor signals a lack of cleanliness. It may merely be the result of not using deodorant.

- Rethink your assumptions about someone's dress. What might be the reason behind the choice of apparel?

- Learn about the meaning that others attach to dress and appearance by asking about it in a nonjudgmental way.

- Make sure you explain the business reasons for any dress code regulations.

Food and Eating Habits

One of the most obvious and widely appreciated aspects of cultural differences relates to food. Cultures differ not only in their cuisines but also in their habits and rules of etiquette for eating, as well as in their beliefs about food's role in health and healing. Often those beliefs and practices may seem more foreign than the exotic spices or unusual ingredients of a particular dish. For example, it may be surprising to learn that in mainland China hospitals have no kitchens or food service departments. Families are responsible for feeding their loved ones in the hospital and bring portable woks and the ingredients to prepare meals each day.

Concepts about hot and cold foods in Asia and Mexico prescribe the foods and the temperature of liquids that are needed for recovery from illness. In China, for example, certain diseases are seen as the result of excess heat or cold. Diarrhea and sore throat result from too much heat, while anemia, nausea, and influenza result from an excess of cold. Illnesses in either category are then treated with food from the opposite classification.[4] Many Asian women recovering from childbirth, which they see as a "cold" experience, desire warm liquids, not the ice water usually provided in U.S. hospitals.[5]

Just as you may be familiar with the "feed a cold, starve a fever" dictum or the often-recommended chicken soup remedy, other cultures have belief systems around the healing properties of certain foods. Family members may bring homemade dishes, such as the pig feet stew brought to a second-generation Chinese American physician after the birth of her child. Her Hawaiian-born aunt had prepared it for her because it was believed to reduce the duration of bleeding after birth.[6]

Religious beliefs also guide food preferences, both for staff and patients. Devout Muslims eat no pork. Jews adhering to Kosher food laws eat only food prepared according to Kosher guidelines, avoiding pork, shellfish, and the mixing of meat and dairy products.

Seventh Day Adventists, as well as many others for nonreligious reasons, eat a vegetarian diet.

Becoming aware of these preferences and honoring them gives a very tangible sign of respect to individuals whose practices may diverge from the norm. One urban children's hospital gave a lovely going-away party for its director of nursing, an Orthodox Jew. By having food prepared by a Kosher catering company they not only honored her but demonstrated their respect for diversity.

Suggestions Regarding Food and Eating Habits

- Learn about the food and diet beliefs and practices held by the cultural groups you serve.
- Investigate the reasons behind a patient's refusal of food or liquid.
- Find creative ways to prepare healthy yet culturally preferred foods.
- Offer alternatives that appeal to different groups (such as a choice between potatoes, rice, bread, noodles, tortillas, and pita bread, or the option of a fork or chopsticks).

Time and Time Consciousness

"The early bird gets the worm" and "He who hesitates is lost" are common U.S. expressions that illustrate a strict time consciousness. The *monochronic* orientation, which sees time as a commodity that is saved and spent, and as a line that is divided into segments with schedules, deadlines, and appointments, is generally the orientation of business culture in the United States. There is another perspective on time, however, a *polychronic* one, which views time as a circle within which many things can happen at once. In this view, schedules, appointments, and deadlines are less relevant.

A Canadian clinic serving native people got a clear lesson in this difference. Staff expressed exasperation as patients continued to be late for or miss appointments. Finally a group of clinic users sat down with the staff to deal with this obvious culture clash. Staff explained that appointments were made for the patients' convenience, so they would not have to "waste time" waiting. The Native group explained, however, that they were not concerned about waiting; what they did care about was the emotional state of the clinician who treated them. They did not believe they could be helped or healed by anyone who was angry and upset. They suggested that instead of appointments the clinic should use a first-come, first-served approach so that lateness would not be an issue and staff would not have unmet expectations that led to frustration and anger.

Our orientations about time—whether or not we meet deadlines, arrive on time for appointments, or rush to keep on schedule—not only direct our behavior, they also influence our interpretations of others' behavior. When someone is late, it is often assumed that the tardy individual thinks his time is more valuable than others'. A person who misses a deadline is frequently seen as disorganized, overworked, or underskilled. In addition, the rules regarding time may differ according to position. Physicians may have more leeway to be late than patients or staff. Managers can sometimes walk into meetings late, though staff cannot. Finally, as with all cultural norms and values, there is an upside and a downside to each approach to time. Rigid adherence to time may be efficient, but it may also cause stress, while less attention to time may reduce stress but result in less efficiency.

Suggestions Regarding Time and Time Consciousness

- When time commitments such as deadlines and appointments are necessary, help people to understand the reasons behind them.
- Where possible, make adaptations to suit the time orientations of those you serve.

- Question your assumptions about the meaning of others' behavior regarding time (such as tardiness, promptness, and demands).

Relationships

Who do you consider family? Is it nuclear or an extended group? How do you address older family members, by first name or by honorary title such as Auntie? What do you consider your responsibility to other family members?

Your answers to these questions will depend on your cultural software. Although family is the fundamental unit in most societies, how it is defined and what the reciprocal responsibilities are within it are different in each society. In groups such as Latinos, Armenians, and Gypsies it is common for large, extended, intergenerational family groups to visit patients or for a number of people to accompany an individual to an appointment. Accommodations for larger groups may call for larger waiting rooms and lounges, extended visiting hours, and children's play areas. One hospital in Glendale, California, a city that is home to one of the largest communities of Armenians outside of their homeland, had a clever response to this cultural factor. The hospital took empty patient rooms that had resulted from a lowered census and converted them into guest rooms for family members who wanted to stay near their loved one during the duration of treatment. That decision demonstrated cultural sensitivity, generated revenue, and became a marketing asset for the hospital.

At a nephrology nurses conference, one of the participants related an incident that illustrated the role of family. A nurse had called a patient waiting for a kidney transplant to let her know that an available match had been located and that the patient would need to come in immediately to prepare for the procedure. The husband, who had answered the phone, replied that his wife was unavailable because they were having a big family get-together for which she was preparing and cooking. Although he may not have understood the difficulty in obtaining organs or the small window of time available, he was clear about his priority on family.

In another case, nurses complained to the patient services representative about the demanding behavior of an Iranian patient's family member. In their eyes this family member had overstepped her bounds, interfering in the nurses' care by badgering and berating them. In the family member's eyes, however, she was protecting and taking care of her loved one.

Suggestions Regarding Relationships

- Recognize that having family nearby is a support and aid to healing for many people.
- Ask the patient if there is anyone he or she would like to confer with in making a decision.
- Show respect by acknowledging family members and by addressing the eldest person first.
- Wherever possible make accommodations for family groups to visit, wait, and confer.

Values and Norms

Values form the moral compass of our lives, and they are acted out in the norms or rules of behavior by which we live. They help us to make everyday decisions, yet we rarely question them unless we face a moral dilemma, a situation in which two values or rules conflict. What would you do if you wanted to do something that conflicted with the wishes of your family? When asked this question, Japanese women who were bilingual (they spoke Japanese and English) were asked to respond in both languages. In Japanese they replied, "It is a time of great unhappiness." In English, however, they said, "I'd do what I want."[7] Apparent in these very different responses are the value differences between the two cultures. One culture emphasizes the individual, the other emphasizes the group. This dichotomy between individualism and collectivism is only one of many value differences among cultures. A collectivist orientation can be seen when a patient refuses treatment that would be a burden on loved ones or when staff members find it embarrassing to be singled out for praise. An individualistic orientation is seen when patients ask about their rights or when staff members assert themselves at meetings.

Another values difference relates to balance between tasks and relationships, that is, whether a culture focuses more on accomplishing tasks or on building relationships. In relationship-oriented cultures, task accomplishment is stymied until people build trust and comfort with one another. In those that are task oriented, spending time on relationships may feel like small talk that wastes time. Conversely, a task emphasis may be seen as cold, aloof, and untrustworthy by those who need a personal bond before jumping into a project, an examination, or a treatment.

In one long-term care facility, Filipino staff used to a more relationship-oriented approach were so put off by their task-oriented new administrator that they labeled her racist. She was appalled and hurt by their attack on her character and felt unjustly accused. Assumptions and defensiveness escalated on both sides. The administrator continued to focus on what she thought was making things better by improving procedures, updating systems, and improving skills to streamline operations. To the staff, however, her "improvements" did not make things better at all. They felt overlooked and undervalued as human beings because she spent virtually no time getting to know them and building rapport before getting down to brass tacks. To them she appeared cold, uncaring, and inhuman. Without an understanding of the cultural difference inherent in their approaches and expectations of each other, both parties felt disrespected and devalued.

Another values disparity has to do with the way individuals deal with conflict. Some cultures prefer an up-front, direct, and tell-it-like-it-is style of confrontation. Others find such directness upsetting and prefer a low-key, behind-the-scenes, face-saving way to restore harmony and maintain smooth relations. This difference between two registered nurses in one hospital escalated to an incident of major proportions when a conflict arose between them. These two RNs had very different responses based on their divergent cultural programming. The African American nurse responded with a direct, up-front, let's-get-this-out-in-the-open-and-talk-about-it style. Her Filipina colleague, desiring harmony and smooth relationships, found the open confrontation highly tension producing. She continued to walk away rather than discuss the difficulty, but she was followed by her counterpart, who felt that patient care would be impaired unless they could deal with the problem and come to some resolution. Finally, the Filipina nurse, overwhelmed by the tension, turned and confronted her colleague, telling her that if she took another step closer she would hit her. Both nurses filed a grievance and both claimed to have been physically threatened. Perhaps this unnecessary escalation could have been prevented if each had understood the cultural differences at work.

Suggestions Regarding Values and Norms

- Recognize that culturally related value differences may underlie reactions such as resistance, foot-dragging, or lack of follow-through.

- Investigate the preferences of your coworkers, staff, and patients. See if you can increase your flexibility to accommodate and work with their values.

- Help others understand your values and preferences. The more they understand you, the easier it will be for them to work effectively with you.

- Consider the downside of your values and preferences as well as the upside of those held dear by others.

Beliefs and Attitudes

Expectations about gender roles, specifically the position of women, attitudes toward authority and social order, and the influence of religion constitute another category of cultural teachings. Preference for either a hierarchical system of order or a more egalitarian one influences both staff and patients. Whether an employee takes the initiative to make suggestions and point up problems or expects the boss to direct and the employee to follow his or her lead depends on this cultural aspect. This difference also has an impact on how a patient interacts with a physician—as a partner with whom to collaborate on a joint mission or as an authority figure whose direction is to be followed.

Beliefs about social order also direct the roles of men and women and prescribe appropriate behaviors for each, both inside and outside the home. For example, marketing research among Latinos demonstrates that while males dominate in some arenas, women generally make decisions regarding family purchases and finances. Gender role expectations also affect interactions with patients. A female hospital staff member taking a history from an older Middle Eastern male patient was unable to get any information when she got to the section about sexual functioning and behavior. Realizing the reason for the impasse, she asked a male colleague to complete the interview.

Beyond social order are the religious beliefs and concerns of both staff and patients. Individuals in the United States adhere to an increasingly wide array of religions. Employees may want to take off a variety of holidays or days and times of worship. They may dress according to their beliefs, covering their heads or parts of their bodies. Patients' religious faiths also influence their views of illness and suffering, as well as their culture's practices upon a person's death. For example, Muslims require turning the deceased's body to face East and allow only Muslims to touch the body. Other religions require that candles be lit around the departed. Preventing these customs because of a lack of understanding of their purpose or importance to families can cause unwarranted distress as well as lost trust with the community. An example of cross-cultural sensitivity and cooperation was seen when a female chaplain at a Methodist hospital was asked by the family of an Arab Muslim patient to pray with them. She went to her office and found a non-Christian prayer that was helpful in giving solace to the family.

Suggestions Regarding Beliefs and Attitudes

- Do not take slights personally. Understand the cultural components of reactions and behaviors.
- Clearly explain your title and position to gain credibility in interactions.
- Learn about the religious beliefs and practices of the patient groups you serve.
- Make accommodations for special customs, rituals, and practices whenever possible. For example, some organizations with Muslim employees set aside a prayer room for those who pray five times a day.
- Recognize that respect for age is widespread among cultures. Make sure you acknowledge and address older individuals first.

Mental Process and Learning

Not only how we act but also how we think is partially culturally influenced. Some of us are linear, logical thinkers who use a step-by-step sequence and make lists, outlines, charts, and diagrams. Others of us are more lateral and intuitive, using images, drawing word pictures, or mind mapping their ideas. Some people focus on the big picture, others focus on details. Although all of us use some elements of both kinds of thinking, and neither style is better, cultures and individuals generally find one style preferable. Linear thinkers who wonder why a coworker does not get to the point or who are frustrated by a patient's meandering explanation may have come face to face with this difference. Lateral thinkers might feel that their creativity is squelched by a rigid outline or that their ideas are not understood by someone who cannot follow an explanation without a flowchart.

Another significant difference in mental processes relates to what Rotter has termed *locus of control*,[8] that is, whether or not we consider the events of our lives to be within our control. Those who believe that they have achieved what they have in life because of their hard work, perseverance, and skill are internal in their locus of control orientation. At the other end of the spectrum are those with an external orientation, who believe that their life situation is the result of luck, fate, and factors outside their control. These differences figure into both staff and patient behaviors. Staff whose orientation is more external may have a difficult time understanding the importance of performance evaluations, for example. Their view might be, "I'll get a good evaluation if I'm lucky enough to have a nice supervisor. If I've got a bad supervisor, I'll get a bad review." Those with an internal orientation, conversely, may feel responsibility even for things over which they have no control.

Patients whose orientations are external may have difficulty adhering to treatment regimens and seeing the consequences of not following directions. They live in the present, not focusing on a future that they feel they do not control. A case in point is that of Elizabeth Ortiz de Valdez's claim that Latinos are generally nonlinear and think more about the past and present than about future consequences. Knowing this indicates that a different strategy is needed regarding prevention. Ortiz de Valdez has found that more successful than focusing on future benefits is emphasizing how a particular regimen is good for the patient in the present and how following it helps the patient to have energy and power now.

Suggestions Regarding Mental Processes and Learning

- Use different methods of explaining, perhaps a story or anecdote, as well as bulleted points.

- Discover the locus-of-control orientation of the person you are dealing with, then make points that appeal to his or her viewpoint.

- Recognize that a patient's not following through may not be a sign of resistance or defiance. It may instead represent a lack of understanding of the treatment's importance or its consequences.

- Expand your own thinking style. Experiment with working in your nondominant mode, for example, visualizing rather than making an outline.

Work Habits and Practices

The place of work in life, the status of work, and who is supposed to do what kind of work are also aspects of cultural influence. Some staff would consider certain kinds of work demeaning. For example, although some would consider working with one's hands to be honest work, others would consider it beneath their dignity. Workers are classified in many ways, blue or white collar, exempt or nonexempt, trade or professional, and so on. We also have expectations about rewards and promotions based on our views about work. For some, upward mobility and increase in pay come from achievement and competence. Others expect it because of seniority or connections. Finally, some find satisfaction in the work itself, getting meaning and fulfillment from their labor, while others see work as only a means to an end, a way to pay the bills and get a vacation, benefits, and pension. These differing views of work play a great role in motivation, commitment, and productivity.

Suggestions Regarding Work Habits and Practices

- Recognize that others' views of work and of its place in life may be different from yours.

- Identify others' motivations so you can emphasize the benefits that matter to them.

- Explain the reasons for tasks, especially those that people may resist.

- Make sure that the criteria for rewards and promotions are clear, equitable, and appropriate.

Table 3.1. delineates the main differences in each of the ten aspects of cultural programming.

Questioning and Expanding Your Own Assumptions

Although no one can ever learn all the cultural variations on a theme, once you begin to understand the range of differences you have taken a critical step. Questioning your own interpretations and not assuming they are universal is essential. Then you need to begin to consider alternative meanings and interpretations. Talking with others who have had experience with cultural differences is one way to expand your thinking.

For example, focus on those behaviors that are particularly difficult or frustrating to you. These hot buttons can create serious obstacles in your interactions unless you find some effective ways of dealing with them. Can you see the behavior in a different light? For example, the patient who arrives late may have a different time orientation, may depend on public transportation, may have lost his watch, or may be lazy. The coworker who spends much time in small talk may need to establish a relationship connection before engaging in a task, may be nervous and uncomfortable, or may be unaware of the tight time frame of a project.

Once you see a range of meanings, you can determine more productive responses on your part. The more you learn to question your own assumptions, discover alternative explanations, and expand your repertoire of responses, the more effective you will be in dealing with patients and coworkers, no matter what their cultural software.

TABLE 3.1 Comparing Cultural Norms and Values.

Aspects of Culture	U.S. Health Care Culture	Other Cultures
1. Sense of Self and Space	• Informal • Handshake	• Formal • Hugs, bows, handshakes
2. Communication and Language	• Explicit, direct communication • Emphasis on content—meaning found in words	• Implicit, indirect communication • Emphasis on context—meaning found around words
3. Dress and Appearance	• "Dress for success" ideal • Wide range in accepted dress • More casual	• Dress seen as a sign of position, wealth, prestige • Religious rules • More formal
4. Food and Eating Habits	• Eating as a necessity—fast food	• Dining as a social experience • Religious rules
5. Time and Time Consciousness	• Linear and exact time consciousness • Value on promptness • Time = money	• Elastic and relative time consciousness • Time spent on enjoyment of relationships
6. Relationships, Family, Friends	• Focus on nuclear family • Responsibility for self • Value on youth, age seen as handicap	• Focus on extended family • Loyalty and responsibility to family • Age given status and respect

7. Values and Norms	• Individual orientation • Independence • Preference for direct confrontation of conflict • Emphasis on task	• Group orientation • Conformity • Preference for harmony • Emphasis on relationships
8. Beliefs and Attitudes	• Egalitarian • Challenging of authority • Gender equity	• Hierarchical • Respect for authority and social order • Different roles for men and women
9. Mental Processes and Learning Style	• Linear, logical • Problem-solving focus • Internal locus of control • Individuals control their destiny	• Lateral, holistic, simultaneous • Accepting of life's difficulties • External locus of control • Individuals accept their destiny
10. Work Habits and Practices	• Reward based on individual achievement • Work has intrinsic value	• Rewards based on seniority, relationships • Work is a necessity of life

Source: Lee Gardenswartz and Anita Rowe, *Managing Diversity: A Complete Desk Reference and Planning Guide* (Burr Ridge, Ill.: Irwin, 1993), p. 57. Reprinted by permission of *The Western Journal of Medicine.*

4

Achieving Practical Cultural Literacy

Ethnic imprints may lie dormant or be overt, but they become most apparent in time of elemental challenge—in birth, marriage, illness, suffering, and dying. Ethnicity is a force in both the genesis and healing of illness. It contributes to the uniqueness of the experience of illness—the very uniqueness the physician must somehow penetrate, at least in part, if he or she is to heal effectively. It is, as a consequence, a moral obligation of the conscientious healer to comprehend and to empathize to some extent with the cultural identity of those he or she purports to heal.

Edmund Pellegrino, M.D.[1]

Part of what makes the intersection of diversity and health care so fascinating and complicated is the number of variables that shape a person's behavior and beliefs. Cultural literacy is critical to the practitioner trying to deliver good service. This chapter examines an array of cultural factors that are capable of influencing appropriateness of treatment. The information covered ranges from culturally influenced attitudes and viewpoints about illness and death to the patient's relationship with the physician and the role of the family in making decisions regarding treatment.

Factors That Influence Adherence to Norms

It is important not only to understand cultural values but also to consider the factors that help determine a patient's or employee's adherence to those values. All Chinese—or all Salvadorans, all Indians, or all Armenians—do not respond the same way to Western medical practices. Following are some of the factors that influence the level to which people adhere to various norms.

Level of Assimilation

How open immigrants are to U.S. or Western medical protocols is in part determined by their adaptation to the norms of their new home. The degree of assimilation may be influenced by length of time in this country or by what generation a person is. For example, a third-generation Japanese American will be quite different in acculturation than a first- or even second-generation Japanese American. Length of time in the United States is not, however, an absolute determiner of the degree of assimilation. In Miami's Cuban community, for example, where one can fully experience Cuban culture on U.S. soil, residents never need to speak English and rarely need to adapt to American norms unless they choose to. In a case like this, passive resistance to assimilation is rooted in a lack of need. Adaptation as a survival mechanism is not necessary when a community can recreate its norms and structure on foreign soil. Conversely, if an immigrant comes into a new society without the cultural infrastructure of the Cubans in Florida or the Mexicans in Los Angeles, the need for assimilation will be greater, and in all probability lead to adaptation to common U.S. practices in health care and other areas as well.

Historically, each generation of immigrants has adopted more of mainstream culture as time passes and the length of its stay increases. That adaptation happened more quickly at the beginning of the twentieth century than it does now, because at that time becoming "Americanized" was valued to the exclusion of maintaining the traditions and language of one's root culture. Immigration patterns at the end of the twentieth century are far different than were those at the beginning of the century. Today there is a much stronger push by immigrants to maintain their ethnic identity, including language, customs, and celebrations. Because we are in the middle of the latest immigration movement, it is difficult to predict with absolute certainty the impact that slower assimilation will have on health care. Nevertheless, it is valid to suggest that a person's level of assimilation certainly influences his or her response to participation in the system, his or her follow-through on treatment, and his or her perception of excellence regarding care.

Education

Education or its lack, literacy or illiteracy, and intellectual sophistication or conceptual simplicity also indirectly affect attitudes toward illness and wellness, habits of personal investment in one's well being, and definitions of good health care practices. A peasant who comes from the fields of Mexico will have different expectations of a physician than a college professor from Mexico. So, too, will a minimally educated resident of Appalachia have a different relationship to a health care system and its providers than a scientist from Taiwan, a computer engineer from India, or a college-educated resident of a city fifty miles away, for that matter. Education level changes the nature of the discussion between physician and patient. It can also change physician expectations regarding follow-through on treatment, or influence whether treatment is even sought in the first place.

A woman with little or no education will have a very different attitude toward prenatal care than someone who is well educated. A woman who comes from a small village may have no formal knowledge of trimesters, nor care about them. Information about prenatal care and sonograms may seem thoroughly irrelevant at best, and absolutely foreign at worst. In a community where there is little structural education, unless a hospital reaches out with an awareness program that teaches the importance of prenatal care there is a good chance that the community will pay with expensive treatment at the back end of the process rather than benefit from cost-effective preventive medicine at the front end. This is but one example of how education level affects adherence to health care, and thus wellness.

Another impact of education level involves attitudes toward folk medicine or faith healers. There is a valuable role for such medicine and healers to play, and in some cultures they are as significant to the psyche as medication is to the body. As people around the world become global nomads and increase their education through travel experience, they acquire a wider world view and become less ethnocentric. This increased learning exposes some patients to faith healers, making alternative practitioners one more health care option. Whether the healer's education is formal, such as studying physiology and anatomy at a university, or informal—that is, learned at home—it does make a difference in patient knowledge, demands, and needs.

Socioeconomic Level

Like education level, income or class can be the source of a multitude of cultural differences. Wealth, however, can offer opportunity for wide exposure to a variety of countries and experiences. The result is increased sophistication, wide travel, and exposure to various lifestyles, ultimately creating a range of options and expectations regarding everything from the proper role of a woman in society to how or for what one uses health care services. Someone born and reared in the Middle East would undoubtedly have different expectations regarding health care practices, based on culture and religion, than someone born and reared in the United States. Wealthy Saudis, however, will likely have been educated in different parts of the Western world at some point and hence be familiar with U.S. health care practices. Poverty in most parts of the world limits access to health care as well as to knowledge of a variety of treatment options. These two ends of the socioeconomic spectrum, affluence and poverty, continue to illustrate the difference that income can make in one's health care expectations and experience, both directly, by influencing the care for which one can pay, and indirectly, by affecting the range of health care practices to which one is exposed.

Geographic Location

Geographic location has already been mentioned but we would like to give a few specific illustrations of how it can affect health care treatment and practices. Within countries there are subcultures influenced by urban and rural environments; among countries there are first-world and third-world milieus; and throughout the world there are climatic differences that influence what illnesses people contract—everything from tuberculosis to allergies, AIDS, and other viruses. Eating habits are another outcome of geography that have serious implications. Southern fried chicken differs considerably from California nouvelle cuisine, and traditional fast food, which proliferates across the United States, is certainly different from an Asian diet of rice, vegetables, and fish. How we eat has consequences for weight, obesity, blood pressure, cholesterol levels, and other health conditions. In countries where food and resources are plentiful, obesity with its attendant cardiovascular issues can be a severe problem, whereas in the poorest parts of Africa, malnutrition forces physicians to look at the physical, emotional, and intellectual ravages of hunger.

Geographic location may be a subtle diversity-related issue that influences adherence to Western health care practices, but it does make a difference. The question for you to explore is what influence it, or any of these other factors, has on your patient population. The rest of the chapter should help provide some answers.

Definition and Perception of Illness and Health

One cannot look at the definition and perceptions of health and illness without focusing on two major areas. The first area is the significantly different definitions, interpretations, and approaches toward illness that exist in Western and non-Western societies, and the second area is the stigma and shame attached to some illnesses on the basis of these perceptions.

Physicians trained in Western medicine view disease, for the most part, as a pathology, an abnormality, or a deviation from clinical norms. Illness, conversely, is the way a person interprets his or her experience, influenced in part by cultural categories and in part by social relations.[2] Illness is the human experience of sickness and it is shaped by cultural factors that influence how we view, describe, and talk about the process of not feeling good.

The roots of one's view of illness lie in a complex of familial, social, and cultural interaction.[3] Because illness is so strongly shaped by a tangled interweaving of these systems, the definition of illness is marked by variations across many lines, such as class, religion, age, and ethnicity. How we describe health problems, the kind of treatment we receive, and how long we receive it are all affected by our cultural beliefs.

Western medicine generally focuses on identifying, isolating, then trying to change, control, or destroy the agents of disease. Physicians trained in the West look for a symptom, try to find the underlying cause, then diagnose and prescribe. Prescriptions usually consist of either medication or surgery. Western medicine emphasizes primarily biological rather than psychological influences, and relies heavily on tests, analysis, and technology.

Chinese culture demonstrates a different view. As with many other Asian cultures, balance and harmony are critical. The Chinese physician does not desire isolating a symptom but rather strives to organize symptoms into comprehensible patterns of disharmony. The aim of traditional Chinese medical treatment is to balance these configurations and restore harmony. That harmony can be seen in something as fundamental as not isolating physiological symptoms but rather combining the physiological and the psychological.[4]

A little different from Chinese culture is the Latino perspective on health and illness. This view is holistic in the sense that it perceives that there are many causes of and treatments for illness, and many avenues for maintaining health. The causes tend to fall into three categories: *emotional state*, such as feelings of embarrassment, envy, anger, and worry; *environmental conditions*, such as smog, germs, and poverty; and *supernatural causes*, such as bad spirits, bad luck, or enemies whose envy causes harm.[5]

No matter how illness is perceived, the remedies that work best are those that combine traditional medicine with some nods to cultural appreciation and use some of the folk rituals that aid healing. Said a little differently, culture shapes how a disease is perceived, labeled, and defined. How a person from a different culture understands or sees his illness may, at worst from a Western standpoint, inhibit proper treatment. Illness takes into account social interpretations and in that way stigma becomes a critical variable that shapes treatment. Following are a few examples of conditions that carry stigma:

- In countries as varied as Chile, Kuwait, and Ethiopia it is believed that epilepsy is caused by possession or witchcraft. The epileptic is devalued.[6]

- Some African Americans perceive that when gastrointestinal disorders cannot be cured by Western medicine the condition may be caused by witchcraft or voodoo. This view is just a variation on a theme from superstitions that exist in Anglo culture.[7]

- Probably the most visible example of stigma is that attached to HIV and AIDS in the United States because of the wide belief that people who get it do so by using drugs or by being gay, which in some quarters is viewed pejoratively. No matter how often examples are cited of AIDS as also a heterosexual disease, which people can contract, for example, through a blood transfusion, as did noted AIDS activist Elizabeth Glazer, the stigma and devaluation still exist.

Stigma can add harm to an already painful situation. In numerous studies that highlight various conditions, some people affected with certain diseases become isolated, then traumatized. Others, however, take a more defiant approach. They form support groups and wear their stigma as a badge of honor. Dwayne C. Turner, currently research associate with the University of California Los Angeles Department of Family Medicine and School of Public Health, illustrates the complexity of stigma in an example he shared about an outpatient clinic that Los Angeles County decided to open for AIDS patients. Some of the members wanted the clinic to have AIDS in the name as a way to indicate that they were not ashamed, but many of the Hispanics involved said that if AIDS were part of the name, people in their community would not use the clinic because of the stigma attached by their community. In the end, the concerns of the Hispanic group carried the day.[8] Ultimately the group's pragmatism and desire to serve a large number of people won out over their sense of indignation at being stigmatized.

Even a disease such as cancer, which is no longer loaded with the negative social weight that AIDS currently is, is not immune from stigma. In Japan, mentioning cancer is taboo. The Japanese perceive it as an automatic death sentence. Family members as well as the patient give up any hope of survival upon hearing a cancer diagnosis, and the best coping mechanism appears to be lack of acknowledgment. An example from the "art imitates life" file was the airing of an episode of the CBS medical show *Chicago Hope* with exactly this theme. The brilliance of that particular program was that it clearly crystallized Japanese stigma about the disease, as well as the conflict in cultural norms about how to handle it. The story involved a Japanese family—a husband, wife, and daughter.

The husband was told that his wife had cancer. He was adamant about not telling her because of the shame she would feel and because it is viewed as a death sentence. He was very clear with the two American physicians that his wife should not know. When he left the two doctors, they quarreled. The female physician espoused the view that it is the patient's right to know and the doctor's moral responsibility to tell her. The male doctor was equally adamant about respecting the cultural norms of the patient. In the equivalent of a Shakespearean tragedy involving mixed signals and good attempts gone awry, the male doctor told the patient what her chemotherapy and radiation schedule was because he assumed that the other doctor had already told the patient the truth about her cancer. In fact, she had not, rather she had decided to honor the husband's request. The patient's face registered little to the male doctor, but when the female physician paid the patient a visit later, the patient conveyed her shame and devastation. She said to the physician, "The radiologist could have made a mistake, couldn't he?" The two women just stared at each other, tacitly agreeing to deny the true medical condition. What they did not say spoke volumes about culture clash, and about reconciliation. Their silent collusion to agree that the radiologist erred gave this woman back her dignity and minimized her shame. Although this particular story is a Hollywood tale, it offers a rich reflection of the real-life ethical and cultural dilemmas that occur between doctors and patients, as well as the need to adjust treatment prescriptions based on perceptions of disease and illness.

Key Cultural Values Affecting Care

To fully appreciate the role of culture in shaping a person's relationship to medical care, we need to explore five core values. Once a health care provider understands how these five values fundamentally influence perceptions about all aspects of health care delivery, any practitioner can adapt his or her expectations, the communication process, and the entire delivery of services accordingly. Issues of *status, privacy, fatalism, emphasis on individual or group,* and *access to information* are central to managing the care of every patient. What differs among patients is how individuals interact with each of these concepts. As you consider these values, think about your own patients and coworkers.

Status

All cultures bestow status in some way. The primary questions for health care providers are (1) By what criteria is status demonstrated? and (2) What difference does status make in employee or patient interactions?

In Western cultures, certainly in the United States, status is more fluid than in hierarchical cultures, where stature is given immediately according to gender (male), family name, position in family (oldest male), or title or position. *Professor, doctor,* and *president* all convey high status in the Middle East, Mexico, South America, and the Pacific Rim and Asian countries. In the United States, however, although a name like Rockefeller or Roosevelt has historically had a certain cachet, status is more often given for accomplishment earned by the individual. Michael Jordan, Tiger Woods, Steven Spielberg, Frank Gehry, and Nobel Prize winners are all given status because of what they have accomplished by the strength of their own gifts and talents. Age is not a major determiner of status in the United States, although getting older has less positive value than being young.

When working with patients from cultures in which status is conferred according to, for example, gender, title, birth order, or class, a health care provider should

- Seek out the oldest male in the group when discussing treatment options or giving information.
- Expect high-status people within the patient's family or support group to be very involved in decisions about health care treatment and options.

- Obtain the services of an interpreter, when needed, who has at least equal status to the patient.
- Recognize that any physician will automatically be granted status and treated deferentially. Autocratic decisions about a patient's welfare are often preferred over a physician-patient partnership.
- Expect that women, partly because of status and partly due to privacy issues, might ostensibly exert less influence on their treatment decisions than the men in their lives.

The savvy health care professional will not judge or evaluate whether he or she likes the status criteria of a particular patient's culture. The smart, effective practitioner pays attention and understands that knowledge about status makes the information work for him and can be leveraged to develop a relationship.

If an employee is from a hierarchical culture, how might he or she view

- Challenging a boss?
- Speaking up in meetings?
- Taking the initiative to volunteer for extra assignments?
- Being assertive on his or her own behalf in confronting potential problems?

The employee's concept of status would have an impact on every issue just mentioned. The likelihood is that an employee from a culture where status is given by title, age, or position in an organization will have a difficult time in an egalitarian organization that respects assertion and initiative.

Privacy

One of the sensitive issues in health care is privacy. For the purposes of our discussion we do not mean the confidentiality of computerized medical information. Rather, we are talking about personal privacy. It is not uncommon for people to be shy or modest, particularly when procedures involve disrobing, being examined, or discussing bodily functions with people who are not part of our most trusted, intimate group. Interviews and literature about cross-cultural health care indicate that patients' comfort often increases when they deal with a physician or nurse practitioner of the same sex as themselves. Doing so would help women who have immigrated from Japan or Mexico, for example, to feel a little more comfortable getting a breast examination.

A certain degree of awkwardness exists for many patients in a clinical setting. But that discomfort is exacerbated in some cultures. As a health care practitioner, think about ways to increase trust and feelings of safety. Do not take it personally when patients are reluctant to answer questions that they think are intrusive and too personal. Find a way to get what you need in a less invasive way. Even changing your request for information from a question to a statement that begins with "Tell me" or "Describe" is a subtle but welcome shift. Speaking in tones that convey patience, understanding, and sensitivity is important. Recognize that soliciting the help of extended family members who may function as both cultural and family interpreters is a two-sided coin. On the one hand, the patient may feel safer; on the other hand, he or she may be more reluctant to divulge personal information. Building a good relationship with a patient's spouse, parents, or whomever accompanies the patient can help convey a tacit sense of trust. Most of all, recognize privacy as an issue, and acknowledge that standards around privacy differ. Honoring people's sense of modesty with patience and sensitivity and learning as much as possible about the cultures you serve is helpful. If you can find someone who is bicultural, an individual who functions comfortably in two worlds, get from him or her as many suggestions as possible for overcoming discomfort around privacy issues in delivering the health care that any excellent provider wants to offer.

If an employee is from a culture in which privacy is a prime value, how likely will he or she be to

- Share any personal issue that might affect his or her commitment to work?

- Share a response to an idea discussed in a meeting or share feelings about something that happened at work?

- Build trust in the meet-you-today-trust-you-tomorrow attitude that many U.S.-born employees may be used to?

People from these cultures will build relationships very slowly, and earning their trust will take a long time. This does not mean that these people are cold, aloof, or indifferent. It simply means that they are more private and reserved than other people. Coworkers can come to learn and respect the process of trust building and giving people space.

Fatalism

The concept of locus of control, mentioned in Chapter Three, is central in all cultures and looks at the question of who is responsible for an individual's fate. This concept is an interesting factor that plays itself out in all areas of life. To reiterate, an *external* locus of control figures very prominently in the thinking of, for example, Latin and Middle Eastern cultures. It presumes that what happens to people in life is outside their control and that, rather, what happens to people is fate, God's will, or destiny. The belief here is that the individual can do little to change his or her fate. It has been predetermined. The counterpoint to this perspective is an *internal* locus of control, which is compatible with the rugged individualism prevalent in the United States. This view suggests that what happens to a person is strongly influenced by his or her own actions and choices. True, there are natural disasters everywhere, such as earthquakes, fires, and floods. But the concept of an internal locus of control emphasizes that an individual has control over not only where he chooses to live but also how he earthquake-proofs his home, clears the brush and builds a fire-retardant roof, or builds levies to mitigate flood problems. People with an internal locus of control may not always be able to avoid disaster, but they do not just abandon themselves to the fates either. They do their best to control their environment.

These two contrasting world views have a significant impact on a patient's relationship to health care. For example

- When Andy Grove, CEO of Intel, found out that he had prostate cancer, he was on the Cover of *Fortune* magazine— hardly a private way to handle it—touting the use of the Internet as a way to seek maximum information from top medical experts and become very involved in one's own treatment. He was leaving nothing to chance.

- Nurses in various communities have shared with us that Latina patients are more likely than European American women to believe that there is nothing they can do about cancer.

- In Japan, cancer is often considered a predetermined death sentence and so not even acknowledged.

External locus of control may ultimately change and evolve. The longer a Latino family acculturates to Western norms, or as they increase their education and economic viability, the greater is the chance that female family members will get Pap smears, do breast self-exams, and seek prenatal care. Locus of control, as with all cultural values, is not discreet. It spills over into many categories.

If an employee has an external locus of control, how might he or she

- Demonstrate initiative?
- View the goal-planning process?
- Interpret opportunities for promotion and advancement?

External locus of control can be a tough employee behavior to work with for managers and supervisors who are strongly action oriented. Not an indication of laziness or lack of initiative, it comes from the belief that God does provide, and that what is meant to be will be.

Emphasis on Individual or Group

In this country where cowboys settled the Wild West and John Wayne was king of the terrain, the individualistic culture still rides high. When it comes to health care decisions, the individual generally rules. For the most part, the United States still allows a woman to decide, by herself if she would like to, whether or not she will carry a baby to term. And in many of the various populations in this country, particularly European American and African American, there is a strong sense to not burden the family if one is ill or unable to care for oneself. Contrast care of our elderly with how elderly are cared for in Asian countries. In the United States, one's parent or grandparent gets sent to an extended care facility when the individual can no longer effectively care for the person. In Asia, caring for the elderly seems to be more of a family affair. Long-term care, which is often handled in the home, has an impact on two or three generations of family members. The individual is part of the group, and a sense of duty and loyalty, combined with a collectivist culture, makes putting an individual in any institutional facility unthinkable.

The implications of caring for the elderly are not the only considerations in understanding the differences between group-oriented and individualistic cultures. Group culture necessitates clinics and hospitals providing large waiting rooms for all the extended families who came with patients, and it means that decisions about care and treatment are frequently made by a larger group.

In dealing with staff, balancing these opposing values should play nicely in American culture today because of the emphasis on teams. How can you as an employee or manager structure team work so that individual talent can play out and employees can maintain some autonomy? How can you build the team so that there is a strong sense of the collective good, and so that people do not view decisions and choices through only an individual lens?

Finding a balance between all the values discussed in this section is critical, but finding a balance between the individual and the group is even more crucial. It will show itself day in and day out in the personality of your team.

Access to Information

As much as Americans have complained about the patrician nature of their doctors in controlling the flow of information, the fact is that U.S. caregivers are generally far more forthcoming than their colleagues in other countries. Though such openness—with an emphasis on the right to know—is standard fare for most people born into or acculturated to the norms of medical practice in the United States, it is not necessarily the case in other parts of the world. There are many different Latin cultures, and numerous Asian cultures, with many differences among them, but there is a general practice about what information doctors pass on. Information that is bad news, such as conditions or diseases that are incurable, necessitate not telling the patient. Health care providers in the United States would be smart to tell the family first what the reality is and then take their cues from the family about what to tell the patient. Because there are legal implications and the danger of malpractice suits, it is important to discuss with families the hospital's guidelines on the right of patients to know. Cultural factors need to be part of that discussion.

In a downsizing-rightsizing era that involves rapid change, the right to know is essential because when an employee does not know she fills in with incorrect assumptions, and the organizational culture becomes a less secure place. Therefore the culturally competent manager and employee will

- Not view as worthy of suspicion everyone who is circumspect about what information is shared

- Be careful about when to deliver or when to withhold information that causes shame or stigma

The other cultural values discussed in this section have an enormous amount to do with delivering care to patients. These impacts are presented in Table 4.1.

Non-Western Treatments

Which of these treatments have you used to alleviate pain or restore your health: prayer, amulets, vitamins, narcotics, potions or tonics, herbs, injections, dance, offerings, penance, candles, antibiotics, surgery, leeching or bleeding, massage, manipulation, blood transfusion, medication, chemotherapy, baths or soaks, hot or cold packs, acupuncture or acupressure? Which would you never think of doing? Your answer depends in great part on your culture as well as on your education level and socioeconomic status.

"Wellness has nothing to do with cutting and poisoning," according to Mary Dee Hacker, vice president of Patient Care Services at Children's Hospital of Los Angeles, although surgery and treatments from antibiotics to chemotherapy are commonly prescribed remedies.[9] Healing, a human need since the species has been on the planet, has been pursued over eons using a variety of methods. What is deemed to be successful is often a factor of the era, with various treatments going in and out of fashion over time. From our twentieth-century perspective we might look with horror on leeching, a standard treatment used by physicians in the eighteenth century. Perhaps a century from now health care professionals will look with the same disdain on this era's great reliance on surgery and chemotherapy.

In a diverse community, especially one that is home to newly arrived immigrants, use of home remedies and folk medicine is common. Many patients will continue to use folk remedies or consult

TABLE 4.1 Key Cultural Values and How They Affect Care.

Value	Mainstream U.S. Tendencies	Tendencies in Other Cultures	Implications for Health Care Providers
Status	Earned through accomplishments; given to celebrity; accompanies certain sheepskins, titles, etc.; rarely inherited through family, gender, age, etc.	Given through position in family, title, gender, family heritage, and age.	How decisions get made about treatment and who is involved in decisions are affected by status. In cultures where status is acquired by such things as gender, age, and title, positions must be acknowledged in order to build relationships and trust.
Privacy	On the whole, open to talking about psychological and physiological conditions; even talk shows and newspapers are vehicles for conveying such information.	Respecting privacy and keeping personal matters within the family is a top priority; modesty and shame, particularly for women, also tie into this concept.	A patient's valuing of privacy may make it harder for providers to get necessary information. Relationship building is key, and gaining insight from cultural interpreters can be helpful.
Fatalism	Internal locus of control is dominant. There is a strong sense of control, of shaping one's own destiny, and of accepting responsibility for one's physical health.	External locus of control is more important in many cultures. The sense of fatalism and predestination can be affected by education, socioeconomics, and acculturation. May believe that God's will influences health or illness.	For people who are strong fatalists, the idea that a disease or condition is meant to be, or that it is God's will, may affect attitude toward treatment and prevent intervening on their own behalf.

TABLE 4.1 Key Cultural Values and How They Affect Care, *continued.*

Value	Mainstream U.S. Tendencies	Tendencies in Other Cultures	Implications for Health Care Providers
Individual/ Group	Though there is currently a strong emphasis on teams, there is also a deeply ingrained emphasis on the individual, particularly related to reward structures.	In most cultures, individual will, need, and desire are sublimated to the group. The welfare of the family is seen as paramount.	Care facilities will need bigger waiting rooms for extended families, decisions may be made by a large group, and the patient cannot be considered in isolation.
Access to Information	Right to know is strong; there is a strong sense that information is power. Though some people clearly favor denial and lack of information, most want the straight scoop.	Must take into account perception of the illness and the stigma or shame attached. Is often desirable to withhold information from the patient, particularly when there is a terminal diagnosis.	The health care provider who assumes that full information is wanted could be wrong and could negatively affect the patient's psychological well-being. There is a critical need to learn about the patient. Get clues from family and patient before telling all.

non-Western practitioners such as herbalists or *curanderos* while at the same time seeking help from the Western medical establishment. However, because most patients sense that their folk medicine is not valued by modern-thinking Western health care providers, they may conceal their use of such treatments. It is important for health care professionals to understand these practices so that their prescribed treatment can be adapted to the patient's beliefs and needs, increasing the chances that it will be followed and lead to the success of the healing process. Patricia Walker, a physician who grew up in Southeast Asia, speaks Thai, Lao, and Cambodian, and treats Southeast Asian immigrants in Minnesota, maintains that when she encourages patients to continue seeing a traditional healer, they also come back to her for health care.[10]

Mainstream health organizations are beginning to respond to a growing acceptance among health care providers of alternative medical treatments. A recent article in *The Los Angeles Times* reported that Lifeguard Health Care, a Central and Northern California HMO, will extend benefits to include acupuncture treatment. In addition, the article stated that Oxford Health Plans, an HMO in the Northeast, created a network of chiropractors and acupuncture and homeopathy providers. Members can go directly to these alternative providers. Yoga is also offered as an optional benefit.[11]

Another example of changing Western attitudes are the results of a survey by the John Templeton Foundation and the American Academy of Family Physicians that reported that 55 percent of family doctors use meditation and relaxation techniques with patients. Furthermore, although only 44 percent of doctors learned these techniques in their medical training, 76 percent of male physicians and 85 percent of female physicians believed that such techniques should be part of medical training.[12]

Traditional or folk remedies generally fall into three categories: (1) substances that are ingested, such as herbs and potions; (2) procedures done on the body, such as dermabrasion or acupuncture; and (3) actions the patient can take, such as wearing an amulet or using the services of a shaman. The first two remedies deal with the physical aspects of illness, the last deals with the psychological-spiritual component.

Ingested Substances

The use of medications—both how and from whom they are obtained and what form is preferred—varies across cultures. Prescribed medications may be obtained from pharmacists, herbalists, healers, or on the street in some countries. In many Latin American countries pharmacists can prescribe medicine, and a wider range of medications can be purchased over the counter than in the United States. In Southeast Asia, prescriptions are not written and most medicines, even antibiotics, can be purchased over the counter.[13] Immigrants to the United States may obtain prescribed medicines from relatives or friends in their home country, where they may be cheaper and easier to obtain. Furthermore, the person for whom the medication has been prescribed may share it with other family members.

Other cultural practices in the use of medications may also differ. Southeast Asian patients, for example, may expect to receive medicine at each visit to a Western health care provider, regardless of diagnosis, and will frequently go to another clinic if medicine is not given by the first provider. They also often believe that Western medicine is "hot" and powerful, so they may not take the full dosage. Some Hispanics also may stop taking medication if it does not immediately help, or they may discontinue long-term regimens as soon as they work.[14]

Even in the United States, unprescribed traditional or folk remedies are still widely used. As children some of us were given chicken soup when we were sick, or offered chamomile tea after a chill. Many people still turn to orange juice to ward off colds. These common home remedies for ordinary, run-of-the-mill maladies are typical of the kinds of folk medicine practiced in cultures around the world. For example, according to Lillian S. Lew, expert on Southeast Asian health practices, Southeast Asians commonly use lime and lemon juice, salt, ginger, lemongrass, mint, onions, and garlic for medicinal purposes.[15] Generally the use of these remedies is passed on within families through oral tradition. Substances used vary not only from culture to culture but also from village to village, and even from one family to the next. Beyond the use of home remedies, medicines are dispensed by an herbalist or traditional healer. According to Patricia Walker, those substances that do not contain lead or arsenic may be helpful because of their psychological or placebo effects.[16]

Variations not only in substances but also in the preferred form of administration may be cultural as well. Many prescribed medications can be administered in different forms, such as injections, pills, liquids, and slushes. It is helpful for Western health care practitioners to find out each patient's preference. For example, injections are common in Southeast Asia (Thailand, Vietnam, Cambodia, and so on), hence patients from this area might expect an injection and might not feel adequately treated if none is given,[17] whereas in some parts of the world medicines are given in a drink or slush, so pills or other forms of medication may be less likely to be taken.

Procedures Done on the Body

Massage and chiropractic manipulation continue to be used as forms of treatment in the West; mustard plasters for chest colds may be part of childhood memories for some people; and U.S.-born individuals are increasingly turning to alternatives such as acupuncture, acupressure, and reflexology to alleviate pain and restore health.

Some practices may be less widely understood, however. Dermabrasion, the practice of rubbing coins, which are sometimes heated, on oiled skin to alleviate head or neck pain and other symptoms, is a common treatment among Southeast Asians. The back, neck, head, shoulders, and chest are rubbed, producing a red welt. Another related treatment is cupping, placing a small heated cup usually on the forehead or abdomen. As the cup cools, a negative pressure results, leaving a circular mark on the skin. Moxibustion is another variation, making small superficial burns by touching with incense or putting some combustible material in the skin. This procedure may be used with acupuncture, which involves placing needles in strategic points on the body. Applying medicated paper, pieces of paper soaked in aromatic oils, on the skin is yet another procedure.[18]

Actions the Patient Can Take

Patients may look to rituals, healing ceremonies, and objects worn both to prevent illness and to return one to health. Some older Americans may remember being made to wear cloves of garlic in pouches hanging on strings around their necks during the devastating World War I era influenza epidemic that took thousands of lives. The parents clearly believed that the garlic would prevent their children from being stricken by the often deadly disease. Wearing copper bracelets or crystals are modern versions of the use of objects worn or carried on the body to ward off illness, alleviate pain, or return an individual to health. Some patients may wear amulets, bracelets, or strings around their wrist or waist that they believe to have protective or healing functions. For example, a blue pendant to ward off the evil eye may be worn by Gypsy patients.

Patients may also seek the help of shamans and spiritual healers to deal with their ill health. Such folk healers are believed to have contact with God and/or the supernatural. A small percentage of Mexican Americans and some other Hispanics may go to a *curandero* or *curandera*, some Cubans and Caribbeans may make use of a *santero* or *santera*, and some Puerto Ricans may go to *espiritistas* to intervene with the spiritual world and assist healing. Southeast Asian patients also may seek traditional healers, such as Hmong

Shamans or Cambodian *Kru Khmer*. Laotians who believe that there are thirty-six souls and that surgery is a cause for soul loss have an elaborate ceremony to return the soul to the body after surgery.[19] In addition, among some African Americans from the rural south, belief in magical spells, hexing, and charms to counter "unnatural" illnesses still exists.[20]

The Best of Both Worlds

Western and traditional medicine do not have to be adversaries. In fact, they can work in tandem, complementing each other. An example of cooperation takes place on the Catawba reservation in northern South Carolina. In the Catawba Nation's longhouse, both Dr. David Brady and medicine man John George are respected healers. Their partnership approach goes beyond coexistence and toleration. These two health care professionals share notes on patients and confer on treatment. Their mutual respect is evident in Brady's comment in a recent *Los Angeles Times* article: "We talk about things. John recently came to me and said, 'I have a patient that has a problem and she wants to try this. Will that be OK? I don't want to cross her up on what you're giving her, versus what I'm giving her.'"[21]

Because Brady works more in the clinic and George works more on the reservation, the sharing is built into the system. Patient health histories are done in triplicate, one going to each of the healers and one remaining on file at the clinic. Patients generally go to Brady for checkups and prescriptions and to George for spiritual guidance, but George's monthly sweat lodges help with both physical and mental healing. The mix works well, and Brady says, "What I'd like to see in the future is that some of the Catawba kids who are currently my patients train for medicine. I'd like to see them go off and become M.D.'s and do coyote medicine—that is, mix the medical with the medicine man. . . . When one of them returns and says they've come to replace me, I'll step aside."[22]

Beliefs About Illness, the Body, and Its Functioning

According to Navajo medicine woman Annie Kahn, "What causes sickness? Anything that interferes with living! Being in balance creates healing."[23] Native Americans are not alone in their belief in balance as essential to health. Many Hispanics hold that an individual's sense of *bienestar* (well-being) depends on balance among the emotional, physical, and social arenas and that illness results from experiencing a strong emotional state, such as rage or sadness, which disrupts equilibrium. In addition, many Hispanics believe in the hot/cold theory of disease and treatment, which sees illness as caused when hot and cold are not balanced, and works from the premise that foods and medications cure illness by restoring balance. "Hot" illnesses are cured by "cold" medications and foods, and vice versa. For example, Hispanics who believe a cold is caused by a cold draft would respond better to directions to drink hot teas and soups rather than cold juices.[24]

A similar adherence to the belief in balance is common in many Asian cultures. The concepts of yin/yang and hot/cold are the primary expressions of this belief. Southeast Asians, for example, generally share a belief that there are three classes of illness: physical, metaphysical, and supernatural. *Physical illnesses* are caused by accidents, such as a broken bone or a cut; by eating something bad that causes food poisoning; or by infectious disease, such as malaria or tuberculosis. *Metaphysical illnesses* are those caused by imbalances of yin/yang polarities or hot/cold energies or by emotional excesses. "Hot" illnesses, such as fever or cold sores, come from within the body while "cold" ones are caused when cold gets into the body. In this case, hot and cold are energies or elements in the universe rather than temperatures. *Supernatural illnesses* are those resulting from soul loss or the work of spirits.[25] Shamans or spiritual healers are often called upon to help deal with illnesses in this category.

Among some poor, rural African Americans, illnesses are classified into two categories: natural and unnatural. *Natural illnesses* are those caused by not taking care of the body or by sinful behavior. *Unnatural illnesses* are those that are seen as the work of the devil, witchcraft, magic, or spells. Maintaining health by taking care of the body entails avoiding extremes of heat or cold, being adequately fed, attending to cleanliness, and getting rest and exercise. Breaking rules and not acting "right" spiritually or socially can bring on illness of the unnatural type.

In addition, beliefs about blood are prevalent among this group. Thick and thin, high and low, and clean and dirty blood are common concepts in this belief system. A focus on cleanliness, for example, inside and out, to keep the body free of impurities, can lead to an overuse of laxatives. *High blood* refers to the amount or location of blood in the body, such as a sudden rush of blood to the head, and *low blood* is associated with anemia. This concept can result in misunderstanding, with patients confusing this factor with high and low blood pressure.[26]

In addition to viewing illness as a result of physical and nonphysical factors, patients from other cultures may have different concepts about physiology and may attach different meanings to parts of the body. According to researcher Nikki Katalanos, among Southeast Asians the head is the source and essence of life and generally untouchable. The Lao, for example, believe that disturbing the head causes loss of soul. Direct eye contact is seen as aggressive and many Cambodians believe it can cause illness. The area between the waist and knees is very private and almost never exposed, making physical examinations difficult if not traumatic for some patients. In addition, blood is seen as life's energy force and its loss is thought to be irreversible.[27]

This belief was the source of an upsetting culture clash in one urban children's hospital. A European American doctor treating a critically ill Vietnamese child called for an interpreter because he was having trouble communicating with the child's parents. When the interpreter arrived, she was surprised to find that the parents had a good command of English. The problem, it seemed, was the culture, not the language. They could not understand why the doctor continued to take blood samples every few hours but had still not made a diagnosis. They were fearful that the loss of blood, which they viewed as irreplaceable, was continuing to weaken their already gravely ill child. The physician had tried to explain that he needed the samples to run tests to make an accurate diagnosis. Further, he felt that their resistance questioned his knowledge and authority, and he threatened that if they continued to obstruct his orders he would take himself off the case. Once the interpreter explained the parents' cultural beliefs about blood, he calmed down, allayed their fears, and was then able to continue treatment with their confidence.

Childbirth

This first of life's milestones is dealt with quite differently across the globe. For example, many newcomers to the United States are not used to prenatal checkups. Methods of delivery also differ. Southeast Asian women generally have a short labor (two to four hours) and many prefer to deliver their baby in a squatting position beside the bed. During labor they drink only warm water, and afterward they prefer hot chicken broth.[28]

The National Coalition of Hispanic Health and Human Service Organizations reports that Hispanic women were three times more likely than non-Hispanic white women not to get prenatal care or not to begin it until the third trimester. The report goes on to say that only 60 percent of non-Cuban Hispanics as well as non-Hispanic blacks began prenatal care in the first trimester compared to 80 percent of non-Hispanic whites.[29]

The role of family members also differs. Among Southeast Asians, women often give birth at home with the help of their husbands, who kneel behind them and brace them during labor.[30] Elaine Vandeventer, director of education at Methodist Hospital in Arcadia, California, which serves a high percentage of Asian patients, especially Chinese, gives other insights into the role of family members in childbirth. According to Vandeventer, babies are taken care of by their grandmothers, both the mother's mother and her mother-in-law. She also notes two other differences that have an impact on childbirth. First, because of governmental population control laws in China and the preference for sons, it is not uncommon for Chinese women who can afford the trip to come to the United States to give birth to a prohibited second child. Second, Chinese women may request Cesarean rather than vaginal deliveries and are surprised to find that this is not an elective procedure in U.S. hospitals. Cesareans are favored by these women because they see the procedure as a means of maintaining the ability to please their husbands sexually.[31]

Death and Dying

The definitions of such fundamental concepts as life and death also differ by culture. Is a patient alive when the heart beats but the brain is dead? Should life-support systems be utilized, and if so, for how long? Should medical professionals be allowed to perform an autopsy? Is permitting the harvesting of a deceased loved one's organs for donation considered "right"? Answers to bioethical dilemmas are strongly influenced by a patient's cultural background. According to Barbara Koenig and Jan Gates-Williams, many differences in preference exist. For example, hospice care for terminally ill patients is not universally valued. The emphasis of such care on a peaceful, accepted death in familiar surroundings with family near rests on white middle-class assumptions not shared by, for example, African Americans, who have more negative attitudes toward hospice care.[32]

Another perspective is that of many Chinese immigrants who believe that ghosts inhabit dwellings where someone has died, so they avoid death at home. In fact, death at a property in some Chinese neighborhoods may affect that property's real estate value.[33] Conversely, among Koreans traditional values direct that the patient die at home, with the male head of the family expected to see that this occurs.[34]

What makes understanding preferences sometimes difficult is that a culture often has opposing tenets. According to Chinese tradition, letting nature take its course is preferred, especially if the patient is suffering. In addition, the right to choose death is accepted and one's choice must take into consideration the effects on society. If life-sustaining procedures are a burden on the family, stopping it is likely to be requested. The opposite view, however, that life should be preserved at all cost and that stopping life support interferes with the patient's karma, is also part of Chinese tradition.[35]

Traditional Orthodox Jewish teachings, which are based on belief in the sanctity of life, favor continuing life support measures. Conversely, non-Orthodox Jews may refuse life support, seeing no redeeming features in suffering. In this view, pain and suffering should be alleviated.[36] Most Filipinos and Mexicans who follow the Catholic faith hold that it is morally wrong to encourage death by stopping life support. In addition, among Mexicans enduring an illness is seen as a sign of strength.[37]

Whether or not to resuscitate represents another culturally influenced decision. Differences exist between African Americans and European Americans. The former, often mistrusting of the medical establishment, are less willing to complete forms indicating the patient's desires about life-sustaining treatment. In addition, a study by Koenig and Gates-Williams shows that more African Americans and Hispanics than whites expressed a desire for doctors to keep them alive regardless of how ill they were, while whites desired an end to life-prolonging treatment under certain circumstances.[38] Furthermore, a study comparing elderly people in four cultural groups in Los Angeles reported that 80 percent of Hispanics and Korean Americans believed that life-sustaining machines should never be stopped because there is always a chance for a miracle. Only a third of European Americans held this view. In addition, the study reported that most Korean Americans and Hispanic Americans thought it was harmful to discuss death with the patient.[39]

When dealing with patients and family members about death

and dying, much sensitivity and communication is required. Finding out as much as possible about their views of the sanctity of life, their definition of death, their religious beliefs, and their social-familial support system is crucial.[40] At an urban children's hospital, parents of a critically ill child refused, on religious grounds, treatment that could save their son. Staff got a court order to proceed with the treatment, thereby saving the child's life yet dooming him to spiritual death in the eyes and belief system of the parents. Administration spent many hours counseling staff members and ultimately required only those who could support the hospital's decision to care for the child. As a provider of health care, it is essential to understand that your beliefs, views, and values may be different from those of your patients, and to show respect for theirs, even if you disagree.

Practices upon death also vary widely among cultures. Allowing for cultural and religious rituals is important. For example, many Muslims, upon the imminent death of a loved one, would want to be able to stay in the room and recite the Koran, making these the last words the patient hears. Family might also need to turn the bed so that the deceased faces Mecca. Finally, non-Muslims are not to touch the deceased, so gloves need to be worn.

Autopsies are another arena in which cultural and religious differences may clash. Autopsies are prohibited by Orthodox Judaism. One study also revealed significant differences in the rates of autopsy of Mexican American and Anglo American stillborns and those over forty. The research showed five areas in which the attitudes of the two groups toward autopsy differed, resulting in the disparity in percentages:

1. Mexican Americans viewed the information obtained through autopsies as useless; Anglo Americans saw it as a way to increase scientific knowledge.

2. Mexican Americans saw a before-death request for autopsy as a sign of physician abandonment of the patient; Anglo Americans did not.

3. Mexican Americans focused on the benefit of the autopsy to the family; Anglo Americans saw the benefits to society.

4. Mexican Americans emphasized the importance of keeping the cadaver whole more than Anglo Americans did.

5. Many Anglo Americans believed that the soul leaves the body upon death; many Mexican Americans believed that it remains in the body for several days after death.[41]

Family and Its Role

The strong individualism of U.S. culture may limit who is involved in health care decisions, but patients of other backgrounds may have a different view. What may be seen as interference by those who operate from a more individualistic value base would be seen as loving and supportive involvement by those who come from a more collectivist background. Among such cultures, families are supposed to make the decisions and the patient is spared knowing the unvarnished truth. One son explained, "For us Chinese, we are not used to telling the patient everything, and patients are not used to this either. If you tell them, they can't tolerate it and they will get sicker."[42] In Southeast Asian groups, generally the eldest male will be the decision maker.[43] Among Cambodians, elderly individuals are dependent on their families to provide for them and care for their health. If they have no children in the United States, they are often "adopted" by nieces, nephews, or cousins. The daughter or daughter-in-law is expected to handle their medication and diet.[44]

Mexican Americans usually expect the family to be involved in all aspects of decision making regarding a terminally ill loved one. The father or husband is generally considered the head of the household and the primary decision maker; the wife's input, however, though not obvious, is usually influential.[45] When making decisions about treatment, and about informing the patient, health care providers need to take into account how the patient views his or her role in the process and who he or she expects to be involved in the decision.

Cultural Beliefs About Health, Disease, and Healers

Following is a short summary of health-related norms and preferences of a number of ethnic groups reprinted from the work of Kim Witte and Kelly Morrison.[46] Although you need culture-specific information about the groups you care for and work with, remember to take into account the whole person, to see him or her as a unique individual; do not assume that a particular patient fits the general cultural descriptions of his or her culture.

AFGHAN REFUGEES

Practice indirect communication, avoid saying "no" directly, communicate by stories, extend ritual courtesy between people of differing status, will shop around for doctors, expect injections or pills at medical visits, may not admit to traditional beliefs and practices.

AFRICAN AMERICANS

Classify illness according to "natural" and "unnatural." Combine practical, magical, and religious beliefs. Illness may be viewed as "an attack" on the body and may involve beliefs relating to blood and flow (i.e., blood/flow is too thick, too thin, too much, too little). May seek traditional healers instead of, or in addition to, biomedical help.

CHINESE

May be reluctant to seek physician care. Expect to receive medication at visit and may lack confidence in physician who does not dispense medication. Individual concerns are subordinate to what is best for the whole community or family. Religion is central to beliefs.

EAST INDIANS

Reluctant to disagree [with] or contradict those with high status. May say "yes" even when they do not understand. Multidrug therapy is common and they like colored medication. Injections are popular. The "hand quality" of the physician is important and they may prefer to have their medication handed to them by the physician. Family is involved in patient care. Women and children typically will not visit a physician unaccompanied by a chaperon who will be present during the exam. Reluctant to have blood drawn or to donate blood. Medical pluralism exists, but they may be somewhat resistant to the use of Western medicine.

ETHIOPIANS

Traditional medical beliefs consist of "indigenous magic or religious practices and beliefs."[47] May use both traditional cures and Western biomedicine. Family, friends, and religion are important. Many times physicians are expected to communicate through family members rather than directly with the patient. Concern is with medical diagnosis rather than prognosis. Trust is a major factor in physician-patient relationships. May evaluate a physician in terms of his or her warmth and manners. Most want to be reassured by the physician that they will make it through their medical crisis.

FILIPINOS

Very receptive to modern medicine, yet still retain indigenous disease beliefs. Place a high value on proper social conduct, avoiding unpleasantries, confrontations, and discourtesies. Practice proper respect for authorities. Often delay seeking medical attention. Prefer Filipino practitioners or folk practitioners and value personalism. May be receiving multiple treatments and tak[ing] multiple medications (i.e., herbs and medicinal drugs) at once. Role of family is ultimately important, thus it may help to have a family member or close friend present during the encounter. Often are reserved and overly compliant. Value harmony. Group is more important than the individual.

GYPSIES

Illness is a social experience, with family and friends supporting the sick person. They do not like to be alone. May be expected to consult with older relatives in treatment decisions. Traveling, good luck, cleanliness, and being overweight are all linked with good health. Avoid nongypsies and hospitals but will seek out the "best" medical care. Will try multiple cures for an illness, including nongypsy practitioners, gypsy remedies, and faith healers. Illness can be caused by spirits or the devil.

HISPANICS

May have to seek eldest member of family for treatment consent. Expect authoritarianism, formal friendliness, and respect. Neglecting to shake hands is an insult. May be very respectful, nodding and saying "yes" even if they don't agree, and will avoid directly contradicting physician.

JAMAICANS

Symptoms are believed to be identical to disease, therefore if there are no symptoms, no disease exists. Similarly, treatments are evaluated in terms of how quickly the symptoms disappear. There are specific beliefs about what causes illness (Hippocratic humoral concepts and germ theory), and a treatment must "fit" the illness for it to be used by the patient or considered effective. Self-medication is common.

JAPANESE

Readily report large amounts of information concerning their problems during encounters. Patient and family are often responsible for healing. Poor prognosis should be

communicated to family, not patient. Often seek medication
for a wide array of daily problems and may expect it to be
dispensed in large quantities. Social groups take precedence
over individual needs. Value harmony.

KOREANS

Clients often visit clinics in groups of family or friends.
Expect a relationship of trust (mutual harmony or unity)
between patient and practitioner. May be dissatisfied with
diagnoses that are not the result of laboratory tests, impressed
by diagnostic machinery.

MALAYSIANS

Categorize illnesses according to "usual" and "unusual."
Will seek different healers for different illnesses. Relationship
with healer must be harmonious otherwise treatment will not
be effective. Will seek other healers/practitioners if treatments
do not work or if relationship is not harmonious.

MIEN

Family and religion are central to health beliefs. Expect
medication, and injections are extremely popular, thus
multidrug therapy is common. Traditional healing is common,
and many therapies are related to diet. Believe that you must
understand illness causation before you can effectively treat it.

NAVAJOS

Silence is highly valued, signals respect and attentiveness.
Traditional Navajos prefer to be addressed by kinship titles
(mother, father) rather than names. Value handshaking. May
be offended by being rushed, interrupted, or practitioners not
listening. Have a tendency not to ask questions or confront
others. Expect to take time in their communication and establish rapport, avoid directness. Should avoid speaking of death.

RUSSIAN ÉMIGRÉS

Have trouble understanding the concept of "preventive medicine" because in Russia "you don't think about your health until after you are ill."[48] Possess grand expectations for "American" medicine, to the extent that miracles can occur. Many do not comprehend biological causes of illness because they perceive "macrosocial" causes of illness, such as "war, immigration, political difficulties, and a poor medical system" (Brod and Heurtin-Roberts, 1992, p. 334). Appreciate physician's personal attention and efforts to explain and answer questions.

SOUTHEAST ASIANS

To some, the head is sacred and should not be touched. Similarly, because the feet are the lowliest part of the body, they should not be pointed at the patient because this is seen as an insult. Direct gaze between people of different status is avoided. Many adhere to politeness rules and will agree whether or not they understand, and avoid the use of "no." May delay seeking medical help and expect authoritarianism among physicians.

VIETNAMESE

Religion is central to health beliefs. Believe in both "good" and "evil" spirits. Obligation to family takes priority over self. Place great importance on harmony and maintaining self-control. May appear calm on the outside when actually are very upset. Practice ritual politeness, courtesy, and respect, especially to higher status individuals. Touching another's head and pointing feet toward another should be avoided; women may not shake hands but shaking hands is typically acceptable among men; direct eye gaze is avoided because it signals disrespect. Prefer indirect communication. Accept multiple causes of illness and may combine traditional and

Western medicine. May delay seeking medical attention
because of value placed upon stoicism and endurance.
May be resistant to surgery, and fear loss of blood.

Cultural influences are complex and multifaceted. It is impossible to know all the rules about each specific group. Although this
chapter has demonstrated many culture-specific preferences and
norms, it is not intended as a template. Cultural generalizations
categorize areas of similarity in preferences, norms, and values,
which should not be applied with certainty to each individual.
Therefore, when treating a patient who is from a different background, it is more effective to investigate and check out your
assumptions than to operate on incorrect predictions. Chapter
Five provides more information about conducting such a culturally
competent interview.

Following is a list of tips for caregivers in treating patients from
other cultures:

1. Avoid making judgments about the patient's beliefs and
   practices.

2. Consider analogous beliefs or practices in which you have
   engaged. (For example, although you may not have gone
   to a shaman or faith healer, you may have prayed for the
   health or safety of a loved one.)

3. Ask questions that help you learn about the patient's view
   of his or her condition.

4. Find out what other treatments the patient is using.

5. Ask the patient to bring all medications that he or she is
   using.

6. Explain procedures carefully before an examination,
   especially when they may be embarrassing and/or uncomfortable for the patient. Assure the patient that all attempts will
   be made to preserve modesty.

7. Avoid touching the patient's head unless it is necessary and then explain the reasons before touching.

8. Ask the patient who he or she wants to be involved in discussions about diagnoses, treatment, and prognosis.

9. Ask patients how much they want to be informed and who should receive information if they do not want full disclosure themselves.

Test your own cultural sensitivity by responding to the quiz contained in Exhibit 4.1.

EXHIBIT 4.1 How Culturally Sensitive Are You? A Checklist for Caregivers.

	Very Much	Somewhat	Very Little
1. I know how this patient defines his or her condition or illness and its cause.	❏	❏	❏
2. I know how much information he or she wants about the condition.	❏	❏	❏
3. I know which family members or others the patient wants included in discussions and decisions.	❏	❏	❏
4. I know the patient's and family's wishes regarding life support.	❏	❏	❏
5. I know what other treatments and/ or practitioners the patient uses.	❏	❏	❏
6. I know what medications the patient uses.	❏	❏	❏
7. I know what form of medication the patient prefers.	❏	❏	❏
8. I know the patient's religious and ethical views regarding health, illness, and death.	❏	❏	❏
9. I know about the patient's life history (such as where he or she was born and raised, education, length of time in the United States).	❏	❏	❏
10. I know about the general health beliefs and practices of the patient's culture.	❏	❏	❏
11. I know how the patient views the body and its functioning.	❏	❏	❏
12. I know how the patient views my role as well as his or her expectations of me.	❏	❏	❏

5

Improving Communication in Diverse Environments

Not surprisingly, when asked what aspects of diversity are most challenging on the job, managers and staff alike put language barriers and communication blocks at the top of the list. Much of the work that goes on in health care settings depends on a high level of clear, accurate communication. Critical information is needed from both patients and coworkers, and information must be accurately transmitted to and received by them.

Language

The degree to which a patient or staff member is fluent in English, or any other language you speak, will have a bearing on your interactions. A prime factor affecting this communication is your attitude toward people who speak limited English. How open are you to working with people who speak with accents? How do you feel when people speak with family members or coworkers in their native language while you are working with them? If you are irritated in these situations, consider what it feels like for them. Do you know a second language? How easy is it for you to use, and how confident are you about your effectiveness when using it?

Those whose English is limited often say that they speak their native language when possible because both their explanations and their understandings can be more accurate, and because it is more comfortable. One nurse manager explained this most eloquently. At a diversity training session for hospital managers a discussion about speaking languages other than English on the job began to heat up. The group started to polarize into warring camps. The nurse manager helped to build understanding and bring the group together with her heartfelt comments: "I'm from the Philippines and my native language is Tagalog. However, I understand that English is the language of this hospital and that most patients are frightened if they can't understand what's being said. So I require my nurses to speak English on the floor and in front of patients. However, you can't imagine how stressful it is to have to speak a second language all day in the pressure-filled environment of this hospital. It is such a relief to be able to sink back for a few minutes into the comfort of my native language."

Non-native-speaking individuals, both patients and staff, also often comment that they perceive they are assumed to be less intelligent and less competent as soon as their accent is heard. To understand accents it is helpful to consider how they arise. Language can be likened to a song that has both lyrics and melody. The "lyrics"— the vocabulary, grammar, and syntax—are easier to learn, especially for adults, than the "melody"—the pitch, inflections, and tone of the adopted language. You can help overcome this barrier by paying attention to the sound patterns of the accents you deal with most frequently and by learning the most common substitutions people make. Examples are the interchanging of *sh* and *ch* by native Spanish speakers and the use of *p* for *f* and *s* for *sh* sounds by Filipinos. Remember, too, that even when someone has an extensive vocabulary in an acquired language, word order and the use of articles (*the*, *a*, and *an*), pronouns, and prepositions may be confusing and difficult. In some Slavic languages, for example, there are no articles; hence it may be difficult for a native speaker of a language from this group to use *the*, *a*, and *an* properly. They may say, for example, "I don't want shot." Another frequent confusion occurs when native speakers of Tagalog, which does not have separate masculine and feminine pronouns, use *he* for *she* and vice versa. To build competence in this arena, one progressive organization offers training for employees on developing a "multilingual ear."

Other Aspects of Communication

Although language differences are often cited as the main source of obstacles in multicultural settings, there is much more to communication than language. Variations in cultural "software" are often at the heart of the misunderstanding, frustration, and miscommunication that occurs when people from different backgrounds come together. A number of aspects of interacting and sharing information, besides language, are significantly influenced by culture, including directness, gestures and facial expressions, distance, touch, topics appropriate for discussion, degree of formality, forms of address, balance of relationship and task, pace, and pitch, as well as the relationship factors of priority and status.

Directness

"Spit it out" and "Say what's on your mind" are popular American expressions of the value placed on getting to the point. In languages that depend on subtle contextual cues and that leave it to the listener to infer meaning, as would be the preference in Japanese or Arabic, information is implied rather than stated. Facial expressions, body language, and tone of voice play a much greater role in cultures where people prefer indirect communication and talking around the issue. For example, rather than pointing out that part of a form has missing or incorrect information, indirect communicators might praise the sections that were correctly completed, implying that the incomplete section is a problem.

In another variation, among Hispanics directness in expressing negative feelings or information is discouraged. This taboo may result in a patient's not following treatment procedures, withholding critical information, or terminating medical care.[1]

Differences in preference regarding directness can be particularly frustrating, especially when specific information and answers are needed. A common problem arises when the health care professional asks, "Do you understand?" and the response is a nod or a yes. Individuals from Mexico and much of Asia find it nearly impossible to say no directly because it signals disrespect, can cause loss of face, and makes them feel inadequate. A response such as "Maybe" or "That would be difficult" is probably a polite no. Avoiding yes/no questions by phrasing the inquiry as a multiple choice question is one way around this impasse. For example, you might ask, "Which of these medications have you taken?" rather than "Did you take this one?"

Gestures and Facial Expressions

Another culturally influenced aspect of communication is the demonstration of emotion, such as joy, affection, anger, or upset. Most Koreans, for instance, are taught that laughter and frequent smiling make a person appear unintelligent, so they prefer to wear a serious expression. While Americans widen their eyes to show anger, Chinese people narrow theirs. Vietnamese, conversely, consider anger a personal thing, not to be demonstrated publicly.[2] Smiling and laughter may be signs of embarrassment and confusion on the part of some Asians. Talking with one's hands is more common in southern Europe than in northern Europe. A direct stare by an African American or Arab is not meant as a challenge to your authority, while dropped eyes may be a sign of respect from Latino or Asian patients and coworkers.

Use gestures with care. They may have unintended and sometimes negative meanings in other cultures. Thumbs-up and the OK sign are obscene gestures in parts of South America and the Mediterranean. Pointing with the index finger and beckoning with the hand as a "come here" sign are seen as rude in some cultures, much as snapping one's fingers at someone would be viewed in the United States.

Distance

American culture generally expects people to stand about an arm's length apart when talking in a business situation. Any closer is reserved for more intimate contact or seen as aggression. In the Middle East, however, it is normal for people to stand close enough to feel each other's breath on their faces. Hispanics typically favor closer proximity than do non-Hispanic whites; thus moving away and keeping greater distance might be perceived by Hispanics as aloofness and coldness. In much of Asia, where cities are crowded and space is at a premium, jostling and bumping in public places are not seen as intrusive or inconsiderate and do not require an "Excuse me."

Think about your patients and colleagues and their use of space. Do you sometimes feel crowded or encroached upon? Are there individuals whom you have labeled pushy because they invade your space? Have you sensed that you overstepped an invisible boundary with someone? If so, you may have been dealing with differences in cultural preferences about distance.

When interacting with patients or coworkers who prefer less physical distance, sitting closer and leaning toward them can help. Conversely, when greater distance is preferred, sitting across a desk, counter, or table may help.

Touch

To touch or not to touch is only part of the question. Cultures also have different rules about who can be touched and where. A handshake is generally accepted as a standard greeting in business, yet the kind of handshake that is acceptable differs. In North America it is a hearty grasp, in Mexico it is often a softer hold, and in Asia a soft handshake with the second hand brought up under the first is a sign of friendship and warmth.

For Vietnamese, it is not acceptable to touch strangers, especially for a man to touch a woman, or for a husband to touch his wife in public. Such touching is considered a sign not of affection but of disrespect. Guiding a Vietnamese patient to a room by putting your hand around his or her back would be uncomfortable for the patient and would generally send the wrong message.[3]

Religious rules may also apply. For devout Muslims and Orthodox Jews, touching between men and women in public is not permitted, so a handshake would not be appropriate. Touching the head, even tousling a child's hair as an affectionate gesture, would be considered offensive by many Asians. Individuals will usually let you know their preferences through their behavior. Following the other person's lead is generally a good guideline. If you need to touch someone for purposes of an examination, explain the purpose and the procedure before you begin.

Topics Appropriate for Discussion

Another difference between cultures is apparent in the subjects that are considered appropriate for discussion. Many Asian groups regard feelings as too private to be shared. Latinos generally appreciate inquiries about family members, while most Arabs and Asians would probably find this topic far too personal to discuss in business situations. In helping a group of Arab exchange students fill out forms an American manager was taken aback when the group's cultural liaison explained that the request for mother's maiden name was offensive. Once he understood that the information was considered private, he created a substitute by giving each applicant a code number to place on the form. In social conversations, Filipinos, Arabs, and Vietnamese might find it completely acceptable to ask the price you have paid for something or how much you earn, while most Americans would consider that behavior rude. Even a seemingly innocuous comment on the weather is off limits in the Muslim world, where natural phenomena are viewed as Allah's will, not to be judged by humans.

- This points to another aspect that relates to privacy. To many newcomers, Americans seem naively open. Discussing personal matters outside the family is seen as embarrassing by many cultures, and opening up to someone outside of one's own cultural group is rare. Thoughts, feelings, and problems are kept to oneself in most groups outside the dominant American culture. This difference may have implications when medical problems are stress related or exacerbated by personal or family problems. Keeping all family matters private is a strong code of conduct. For the health care professional who needs personal information, particularly in sensitive areas involving intimate behavior and bodily functions, to complete forms and do workups, it is less intrusive to spend time building trust and getting to know the individual first. Furthermore, if you know that privacy is a value and that getting documentation may be uncomfortable, you can gently explain the reasons for needing this information, and you can conduct the discussion in a soft, unobtrusive tone. All of these techniques may help the patient get beyond the very difficult obstacle of talking to a stranger about personal matters.

An aspect related to self-disclosure is loss of face, important in some manner in all cultures. In Asia, the Middle East, and to some extent Latin America, one's dignity must be preserved at all costs. In fact, death is preferred to loss of face in traditional Japanese culture, hence the ritual suicide, hara-kiri, as a final way to restore honor. Any embarrassment can lead to loss of face, even in the dominant American culture. To be criticized in front of others, publicly snubbed, or fired would be humiliating in most any culture. However, behaviors that we see as harmless can be demeaning to others. Inadvertent slights or unconscious faux pas can cause serious repercussions in intercultural relationships.

Consider the kind of information you need from patients. What kinds of questions seem to cause the most resistance? Could cultural influences be at work here? When asking for information you think might be considered too personal, let the patient know you realize it might be awkward or embarrassing for them to answer your questions. Also explain why the information is necessary and how it will be used. Perhaps there is another way to get the data or a more private place in which to discuss it. There may even be another individual who might be a more acceptable source of information.

Thinking off the cuff, shooting from the hip, and giving an immediate response to questions are difficult for someone raised with a strong cultural preference for privacy. Therefore, brainstorming at meetings might not get much participation from staff reared in other countries. Giving people a chance to think ahead about issues to be discussed or allowing time for staff to write out their ideas before talking about them may help.

Conversely, when it comes to privacy in territory as opposed to thoughts and feelings, Americans are not so open. Much of the rest of the world does not have this emphasis on privacy. Families may sleep in the same room at home, and work spaces may be communal. In Japanese offices, the boss generally does not have a separate office but shares a portion of the work area with employees. Likewise, in public places a new passenger on a bus or train takes a seat next to someone rather than sitting in an unoccupied section. In this country, that behavior would be considered odd at best and threatening at worst.

Degree of Formality

"Let's not stand on ceremony" is a common American response to what many Americans consider "stuffy" formality. Although a casual, easygoing approach may be comfortable for you, your patient or employee may be expecting a more structured interaction. Generally it is best to err on the side of formality, because you can always move toward a more casual approach if it seems appropriate. Keeping a reserved and formal tone by displaying such behaviors as standing or sitting erectly and maintaining a serious expression is a sure way of preserving everyone's dignity.

Forms of Address

A related cultural difference can be seen in norms regarding how people address one another. In the United States, new acquaintances, older individuals, and bosses are commonly called by their first names, yet this is considered impolite and disrespectful in many parts of the world. In most cultures, formal introductions using surnames are expected as a sign of respect for other parties. In some hierarchical cultures, such as Korea, even family members address one another with titles such as elder brother and elder sister. It is generally safest to begin any meeting with formal introductions, giving the titles and positions of staff members or caregivers and addressing patients as Mr., Mrs., Doctor, or Professor. Titles can be an especially important way for female health professionals to build credibility with patients from backgrounds that are less familiar with dealing with women in positions of authority. Use first names only at the other individual's request. This is particularly important in health care, where title and position bring credibility and a sense of security for patients. In addition, because the tone of a relationship is often set at the beginning, if the wrong message is inadvertently sent and disrespect is felt, damage to rapport can be difficult to repair.

Balance of Relationship and Task

In our time-conscious culture, health care professionals may say that they want to spend time with patients but that they cannot afford it. Relationship building is generally a bigger priority in Asian, Latin, and Middle Eastern cultures than in the United States. Whether you are an admissions representative who needs critical information from a patient or family member, a manager who needs to build trust with employees, or a nurse who needs a patient to follow directions, making a human-to-human connection and building rapport is an essential first step.

Finding the balance between task and relationship is key, yet it is a challenging dilemma. If you jump into the task, trying to get information or give directions before you have built any comfort or connection, you are apt to hit a wall. Conversely, if you spend too much time on chitchat before getting down to business, you will find yourself backlogged with unfinished tasks. You may even frustrate the other individual, who may feel that time is being wasted on irrelevant banter. Pay attention to the other individual and the response you are getting to help you find the appropriate balance.

Status

Society, communities, and even families are not egalitarian democracies in most other cultures. There is a definite hierarchy of status in which age, gender, and position determine power and respect. An accepted pecking order exists within families. For example, an older brother has authority over a younger one, a grandmother has matriarch status, or a husband may expect to be included in all of your discussions with his wife. A member of such a family would not think of making a decision without talking it over with the "head of the family."

A case in point illustrates this cultural preference. A young Chinese American professional was seen as the most qualified applicant for a position. The hiring manager was pleased to offer the young man the job and assumed the applicant would immediately accept. He was quite surprised and perplexed to get a very polite, formal letter explaining why the applicant would not accept the position. It seems that the job seeker had decided to honor his father's wish to join the family business. The manager found it hard to understand that a grown man with a college education would not make his own decision independently. Including appropriate family members in discussions with patients and allowing individuals time to talk over decisions with their significant others is important. If you do not know whether this factor is at play, you may need to ask patients who they would like to involve in the discussion or whether time is needed to allow them to confer with others.

Pace

Pace is both an individual and a cultural preference. Some people speak as though they are on fast forward, while others take long pauses between sentences. Individuals from cities tend to be influenced by the hustle and bustle of twenty-four-hour services, traffic jams, and honking horns, while those from rural areas might have learned to be slower paced and less frenetic. Whatever the individual's preference, forty-hour work weeks and limited clinical hours require people to work at a certain pace to be able to serve patients efficiently. Sometimes, however, your pace and that of patients may not match. Some patients may feel an unintended slight if they feel rushed or treated in an abrupt way. Conversely, patients and staff, alike, who have a more relaxed pace may be viewed as lazy, unreliable, or unintelligent.

Pitch

Another difference between cultures is the pitch at which individuals speak and the meaning attached to these distinctions. A higher pitch spoken softly demonstrates politeness by a Japanese woman and is seen as desired when making requests and giving directions in public settings. That same pitch and softness might sound self-effacing and childish to a native English speaker's ear. In another example, a Russian-born supervisor generated disgruntlement among his employees. They complained to the human resources representative that he was always yelling at them and seemed angry. When the HR representative shared this feedback with the supervisor, he was surprised. He responded that he liked his staff and found their work entirely acceptable. It was his low pitch of voice, which sounded gruff and angry to them, that had sent the wrong message.

Suggestions for Health Care Professionals
Regarding Cross-Cultural Communication

- Pay attention to body language, facial expressions, and other behavioral cues. Much information may be found in what is not said.

- Avoid yes/no questions. Ask open-ended questions or ones that give multiple choices. Remember that a nod or yes may mean "Yes, I heard" rather than "Yes, I understand" or "Yes, I agree."

- Consider that smiles and laughter may indicate discomfort or embarrassment. Investigate to identify what is causing the difficulty or confusion.

- Make formal introductions using titles (Mr., Mrs., Ms., Dr., and so on) and surnames. Let the individual take the lead in getting more familiar.

- Greet patients with "Good morning" or "Good afternoon," and when possible, in their language.

- If there is a language barrier, assume confusion. Watch for tangible signs of understanding, such as taking out a driver's license or social security card to get a required number.

- Take your cue from the other person regarding formality, distance, and touch.

- Question your assumptions about the other person's behavior. Expressions and gestures may not mean what you think. Consider what a particular behavior may mean from the other person's point of view.

- Explain the reasons for all information you request or directions you give. Also acknowledge any cultural differences that may present challenges or difficulties.

- Use a soft, gentle tone and maintain an even temperament.

- Spend time cultivating relationships by getting to know patients and coworkers and by establishing comfort before jumping into the task at hand.

- Be open to including patients' family members in discussions and meetings with patients.
- Consider the best way to show respect, perhaps by addressing the "head" of the family or group first.
- Use pictures and diagrams where appropriate. For example, give maps for directions, or show a picture of a social security card or driver's license.
- Pay attention to subtle cues that may tell you an individual's dignity has been wounded.
- Recognize that differences in time consciousness may be cultural and not a sign of laziness or resistance.
- When appointments, deadlines, and schedules are necessary, explain the reasons for them and the consequences of not meeting them.
- Explain the role of promptness in getting good care.
- Do not take others' behavior personally. Remember that the way people from other cultures initially react to you may have less to do with you personally than with factors such as your age or gender.

Assessing Intercultural Hooks That Block Communication

Being culturally literate enough to understand the numerous influences that may affect your patients' and coworkers' behavior is critical to being effective on the job. But understanding these cultural influences is only part of the process. Equally important is understanding your own responses to these behaviors and dealing with the emotions they can trigger. How do you react when someone's behavior does not match your preferences? What if they speak slower than you would like or show no facial expression when you speak to them? How do you feel when they talk on and on, never getting to the point, or when they avoid eye contact? Often emotions such as frustration, irritation, or anger bubble up.

If you are aware of your own behaviors, preferences, and dislikes, you will have less chance of getting hooked or of having your buttons pushed when you encounter some of these norms. To get beyond the irritations you may feel when encountering cultural differences, it is helpful to identify the specific behaviors that bother you. The cross-cultural hook list presented in Exhibit 5.1 will help you do that. What is your reaction to these behaviors? Do you get frustrated, irritated, or upset by the hook? After you have identified what bothers you, you can then look deeper to understand the underlying cultural programming that might be at play. Once you have done that, you can question the knee-jerk assumptions that are producing your emotional response and consider what you might do to overcome such reactions.

Learning About the Cultures You Serve

One way to help overcome these barriers to communication is to become more knowledgeable about some of the cultural factors, the differences in "software," such as those explained in Chapter Three, that may have produced them. If the checklist shows you what you did not know about other cultures and leaves you with a desire to learn more, here are some additional ways to do so.

Ask other employees. One way to find out about another culture's norms is to ask coworkers from that culture to teach you. You will get a better response if you present your request as a search for information rather than as a complaint. When you inquire, choose someone who has some degree of acculturation and ask for specific information such as

- What are the biggest differences between your culture and that of America?

- What are some of the most difficult adjustments you have made since living in the United States?

- How is respect shown in your culture?

EXHIBIT 5.1 Intercultural Hooks That Block Communication.

Directions: Put a check mark next to any of the cross-cultural hooks that could result in frustration or in negative interactions between you and a patient or coworker.

❑ Nodding or saying yes without understanding.

❑ Speaking in a language other than English.

❑ Deferring to others when asked a question.

❑ Refusing to shake hands with women.

❑ Speaking loudly.

❑ Lacking nonverbal feedback (facial expression).

❑ Speaking softly.

❑ Avoiding eye contact.

❑ Smiling and laughing when nothing is humorous.

❑ Giving a soft, limp handshake.

❑ Standing very close when talking.

❑ Speaking with a heavy accent or limited English.

❑ Making small talk and not getting to the point.

❑ Not providing necessary information.

❑ Not taking initiative to ask questions.

❑ Calling or not calling you by your first name.

❑ Discounting or refusing to deal with women.

❑ Speaking in a high-pitched voice.

❑ Asking personal questions.

❑ Using formal titles in addressing people.

❑ Others _____

- What expectations here at the hospital seem to insult or violate the behaviors you were taught as a child?
- How do patients interact with caregivers in your culture?

One African American physician was seen by her colleagues as a role model in this kind of cultural learning. Fascinated about how other cultures view the world, she makes it a point to talk with physicians who are foreign born. Not only does she gather pertinent information through questions such as Are there things I should ask? Should I ask it differently? and Tell me what I should look for, but she also shares with others what she learns.

One caveat here: Do not expect the individual who is your cultural interpreter to be a spokesperson for an entire group, or your only teacher, whether formal or informal, about a particular culture.

Ask friends or acquaintances outside the hospital who are from other cultures. If you don't get enough information from coworkers, ask friends who are from or have had experience with the cultures you are trying to learn about. They can be invaluable cultural interpreters, teaching you about subtle but often important norms that may cause misunderstanding. They are apt to be able to see things biculturally and to give you some interesting insights into the areas of friction you are trying to resolve or avoid. They may also offer suggestions or help you find solutions. One administrator who got many complaints from staff about one cultural group her institution served tried this approach. She called in a college professor of that background, a woman who had been raised in that culture as well as educated in the United States. The information she received from this professor was helpful in two ways. She gained insight into the cultural roots and reasons behind the behaviors that staff found difficult, and she found that her own ability to relate to individuals from that group was almost magically improved. Whether her own attitude had changed or whether the grapevine had spread the news about her interest in understanding more about her clients and their culture, or both, there was greater ease, more openness, and improved rapport between her and her clients.

Tap community resources. Another rich source of information about cultures is community organizations that have been dealing with these differences for a long time. Ethnic associations (such as the Korean Businessmen's Association), social service providers, and refugee resettlement agencies are good sources of information, as are antibias organizations such as the Anti-Defamation League. They may provide publications with concrete answers to your questions, as well as speakers for presentations to staff. Community relations groups make it their business to help various segments of society understand one another. The Los Angeles County Commission on Human Relations, for example, has published a booklet entitled *How to Communicate Better with Clients, Customers and Workers Whose English Is Limited.*

Read about different cultures. Reading nonfiction books such as *Good Neighbors: Communicating with the Mexicans* by John C. Condon, *Considering Filipinos* by Theodore Gochenour, or *Culture and the Clinical Encounter* by Rena C. Gropper, or titles such as *I Know Why the Caged Bird Sings* by Maya Angelou is one way to get information directly. A list of such publications is provided in the Resources section at the back of the book. Another way to get such information is to read fiction that is set in other cultures, for example, *The Kitchen God's Wife* by Amy Tan (China), *Like Water for Chocolate* by Laura Esquivel (Mexico), *Beloved* by Toni Morrison (African American), *Shogun* by James Clavell (Japan), or *The Color of Water* by James McBride (African American).

Observe without judgment. Pay attention to how people behave without making judgments such as "Oh, what poor taste," "It's low class," or "How ignorant." One of the authors' most enlightening learning experiences came from observing, as a doctoral program assignment, parent-child interactions in two cultures, American and Mexican. Watching parents and their children communicate in Los Angeles and in Tecate, Mexico, showed culture in action. Among the many differences, one stood out. American parents were much more verbal, giving directions by telling their children what they wanted them to do. Mexican parents were less verbal but more physical. They would walk over, take their child's hand or pick the child up, and lead him or her. This kind of detached observation may help you understand your patients.

Share in staff meetings what you have learned. Talk about cultural differences at staff and management meetings. Share insights about cultural norms and how to deal with them. Jorge Cherbosque, an intercultural therapist, consultant, and trainer, suggests that you can even form a peer support group with a multicultural configuration. You can then be resources for one another, giving and getting consultation and advice.[4] Using a case study approach by focusing on a specific cultural obstacle at each staff meeting can give you an opportunity to share learnings and come up with solution ideas.

Conduct focus groups. Another way to get information is to organize culture-specific focus groups with diverse community members to get information through group discussions. Questions such as those you might ask your coworkers, listed earlier, might be used. These groups will give you accurate information and dispel some of the incorrect assumptions that may be influencing your treatment of others. For example, in a focus group with Mexicans, organizers were surprised when they learned that although the culture may be male dominated and patriarchal, the woman takes the lead in making most of the decisions about the home and about family finances.

Use employee or customer survey information. Pick up clues from what people tell you or complain about. If patients comment that staff always seem in a hurry, or that they feel rushed, they may be talking about differences in time consciousness or pace. They may also be indicating a need for more time spent on relationship building before getting to the task. Note, however, that cultural differences affect the survey feedback process. For example, in many cultures written questionnaires are less effective than phone calls. Relationship orientation, oral tradition, and formal education are some of the factors influencing this preference.

Experiment with new methods. When we interview health care professionals who are dealing effectively with their pluralistic patients and staffs and ask how they learned to be more effective and adaptive, they invariably say, "Trial and error." If you are experiencing a culture-related block, try a new behavior or a different approach. Then watch to see how it works.

Spend time in other cultures. Immersion in other cultures is a less traditional but very effective way to learn about different norms. This does not mean that you need to take a leave of absence and live in Mexico, the Philippines, or Korea, although that experience would undoubtedly be enlightening for anyone. Rather, you can watch foreign films, tune in to the foreign-language channels on TV, read literature from and about other cultures, and spend time in ethnic communities such as Little Saigon, Chinatown, or Koreatown. One division of the Los Angeles Police Department experimented with a pilot program that gave officers an opportunity to experience living in another culture.

A group of police officers were sent to live in Guadalajara, Mexico, for six weeks. Although this month-and-a-half stint did not give them enough time to become fluent Spanish speakers, the stay did bring some more important results. Upon returning, the officers reported that they now had a much different view of immigrants and a much greater empathy for the problems and issues that exist for people adapting to a new culture.

Getting Your Message Across: Directions and Feedback

It is often necessary to give patients or other staff members information in the form of clear directions and feedback, especially when there are errors in procedures or omissions on forms. Risk of embarrassment and loss of dignity in these interchanges is increased. In addition, others may have communication preferences and styles different from yours. For those whose culture values subtle, less direct communication as well as harmony and saving face, a direct style may cause so much discomfort that they will not hear your message. The following four communication techniques can lower the risk of misunderstanding and hurt feelings, and increase the chances of getting your message across. Using these techniques does not mean you need to abandon your current methods. Rather, you may add these to your repertoire to expand the options from which you can choose. The more options you have, the more effective you can be because you have a better chance of selecting the most appropriate method.

Make observations rather than judgments or evaluations about behaviors and conditions. People from any culture are apt to get defensive when judgments are made. Objective comments on behaviors or conditions have less sting than a judgment or evaluation, which can cause loss of face or defensiveness. Rather than saying, "This is incomplete," you might focus on the specific problems and explain what is needed. "We need both the name of your insurance company and your member number on page two."

Be less direct by using the passive voice. In languages such as Arabic and Spanish, the reflexive and passive forms are frequently used and actions are often not attributed to individuals. In Spanish, for example, one does not say, "I forgot my papers," but rather, "My papers were forgotten to me" (*"Se me olvidaron mis papeles"*).

Learning to do this may take practice because English favors the use of active verbs. However, this can be an especially effective technique to use in interacting with patients who prefer less direct communication. Using the passive voice means making the object the subject of the sentence. For example, instead of telling the patient, "You've made too many mistakes on this form," you could say, "There are some errors on page two of this form."

Be less direct by making comments impersonal; omit the you. You is one of the most powerful words in the English language. Although it grabs attention, it can also accuse and serve as verbal finger-pointing, producing embarrassment, defensiveness, and even shame. Keeping comments impersonal by omitting the *you* can go a long way in reducing this risk. Instead of "You forgot to get the signature of your spouse," you could say, "The signature of your spouse needs to be here."

Be positive; tell what you do want, not what you do not want. "Don't do it that way" sounds like a reprimand no matter what your culture. It upsets people and does not help them to understand what is needed. When you tell an individual how you do want something done, avoid the wrist-slapping emphasis on the mistake. For example, it would be more effective and explicit to say, "Move carts to the side of the doorway while serving patients" rather than "Don't leave carts in the doorway."

Soliciting Information

Health care treatment often requires eliciting extensive and often personal information from patients. Some people will be forthcoming, while others will find the questioning difficult and insensitive. Gathering information of this sort is by nature prying and intrusive to most people, so it is critical to invest time up front to build rapport and put the patient at ease. The tips on relationship building presented earlier in this chapter can be helpful. Using a wide array of questioning strategies, such as the following, can also help, especially with those from cultures that prefer less directness and more privacy.

Open-ended questions. Rather than drilling for specific facts or figures, open-ended questions give the responder more latitude and are especially useful in the early stages of relationship building, when tone setting and comfort building are important. Such questions can be useful throughout the process when you want to get information from a patient. Such questions are designed to help a person explore options and give full descriptions. Some examples of open-ended questions are

- What problems are you having with your health?
- How have you been dealing with this problem?
- What has made you feel better?

Closed-ended questions. Although you need to open discussion and get general feedback, you also need specific, targeted information. Closed-ended questions are designed to narrow responses and get concrete facts. People from less direct cultures may find these questions more difficult and may respond with roundabout answers. You can help elicit more specific responses with questions such as the following:

- Which payment option looks best to you?
- Do you prefer the medication in a pill or a liquid?
- How often have you been taking the pain medication?

Speculative questions. These kinds of questions require the responder to think about possibilities and show vision. In some cultures, however, such as Japanese, these questions are perplexing and difficult. Some examples are

- Who would be able to take care of your children if you needed to be in the hospital for a few days?
- How would you support your family if you had to be out of work for six weeks?
- How could you get to your treatments if you were unable to drive?

"Tell me . . ." statements. Beginning with these words allows you to disguise a question as a statement. This difference is more than just cosmetic. The punctuation switch sets a whole different tone. Some patients may feel defensive when asked questions. This style protects such patients from intrusion while allowing you to get the information you need. Examples are

- Tell me how your husband feels about this procedure.
- Tell me how you were able to pay off your last hospital bill.
- Tell me about your plans for home care when you are released.

"Describe . . ." statements. This method of getting data has the same advantage as "Tell me. . . ." It solicits information without an intrusive style, in a subtle, indirect way. It reduces the perception of being cross-examined. Examples are

- Describe the movements you make in using equipment on the job.
- Describe how your family can help you follow this diet.
- Describe how your son acts after you give him this medication.

These five questioning techniques will help you get beyond cultural barriers, build trust and openness, and get information from patients in a less threatening way.

Demonstrating courtesy and warmth is the best way to roll out the welcome mat. Some patients may have had limited contact with American health care providers, so the impression you make on each patient will be the definitive view he or she has of you and your institution at the beginning. Understanding cultural differences can assist you in creating an environment that helps patients feel welcome. It also enables you to develop rapport and get the information you need as you explain procedures and treatments.

Most important of all, remember that in the high-stress situations common in health care, both you and the patient will fall back on old patterns of response, regardless of how much you know and how hard you try to overcome your programming. The stress of illness, pain, and deadlines makes all of us reactive. Remembering that reality will enable you to be more compassionate and less intimidating as you probe for the information you need to help patients.

Bridging the culture gap in communication is a two-way street. Both sides need to expand their understanding and sensitivity, and both parties need to bend and adapt. The most important questions you can ask yourself are

- What do I need to know or understand about this patient and his or her background, culture, and needs?
- How can I help this patient understand and meet the hospital's needs as well as mine?

Communicating Across Language Barriers

Whether you are explaining a diagnosis to a patient, giving directions to an employee, or getting information from a family member, there will be times when you will be required to overcome language barriers. There may even be a legal mandate for you to communicate accurately regarding safety, such as California law, Title 8, California Code of Regulation, Section 5194(f), which "requires that employers 'convey the information' available on labels on hazardous chemicals to employees."[5] In addition to understanding the cultural factors that underlay preferences and behaviors, you can also help yourself be more effective by taking charge of your attitude and by preparing yourself for the interaction.

Blocked communication is frustrating and disconnecting, but the emotional overlay you bring can exaggerate the difficulty. Getting a handle on your feelings so you can de-escalate the role emotions play is important. First, confront your own assumptions because they are apt to get you into trouble if they remain unchallenged. Are you thinking that others do not want to learn English? Huge enrollments and long waiting lists at English as a Second Language programs for adults shatter this myth. In addition, many immigrants work at subsistence-level jobs that require long hours and leave little time for formal classes. Are you supposing that they know English and just do not want to use it? Think about your own degree of comfort in speaking another language. How easy is it? To make matters more difficult, even when people have learned another language, stress, upset, or worry tend to make them fall back into the ease of a native tongue. Are you thinking that they just do not care? The hierarchical structure of many other cultures coupled with the educational gap that may exist between you and the patient may present class distinctions that can inhibit the patient's ability to initiate conversation or respond to your questions. To help deal with your own emotional state, take time to question your assumptions and try to walk in your patient's shoes before you begin the interaction. Have you ever been somewhere where no one spoke your language? How did it feel? What would have helped you? Remembering these experiences may give you some empathy for the bewilderment that another individual may be feeling.

You can also take charge by preparing yourself using the following guidelines:

Make it visual. Use visual tools, such as pictures, signs, diagrams, and symbols, to get your point across and make yourself clear. Drawings or a model of the body, a picture of a clock, or colored stripes on the floor leading to different parts of the hospital are examples of visuals that can be helpful.

Demonstrate. As a Chinese proverb advises, "I hear and I forget, I see and I remember, I do and I know." The advantage of a demonstration is that it gives you a chance to have the patient perform the task with you observing.

Use the other person's language. Whenever possible, use the other individual's language to communicate. If you have learned some basic words and phrases, incorporate them into your interchange. Even if you do not know a word of the other individual's language, however, you can still use this technique. One nursing home was temporarily stumped when its elderly residents complained that they could not get the mainly Spanish-speaking aides to understand their needs. A short-term solution was created by printing a sheet with the twenty or so most frequent requests written in English in one column and in Spanish in another column. When residents needed something, they would just point to the request in the English column and the aide could read it in the corresponding line in the Spanish column.

Queen of the Valley Hospital in West Covina, a suburb of Los Angeles, devised a similar method. Seeing the demographics of its community change, with a growing percentage of Latino patients, it produced a handy aid for staff, a small booklet entitled *Speedy Spanish for Nursing Personnel*, which has important health care questions and statements written in both English and Spanish along with a phonetic pronunciation guide for English speakers. The booklet is divided into sections such as greetings, basic anatomical terms, patient complaints, surgical prep, and hygiene/ medical assessment, making it easy to turn to the appropriate section to find relevant words and phrases. (The publisher, Baja Books, also publishes *Speedy Spanish for Medical Personnel* and *Speedy Spanish for Physical Therapists*.[6])

Go slowly. Processing information in a nonnative language takes longer. Not only is the vocabulary, especially medical and technical words, often unfamiliar, but grammar and intonation patterns are sometimes new. Give your listener time to let each segment of your message sink in by speaking slowly and leaving time between sentences. Then summarize at the end, reiterating the main points and pulling the message together.

Keep it simple. "It's a slam dunk," "Let me give you a thumbnail sketch," or "Don't throw the baby out with the bathwater" are examples of idiomatic expressions that add color to conversation and are a common part of everyday speech. Yet, for a nonnative speaker who tries to translate them, they make no sense at all. Medical jargon and acronyms would be equally perplexing. Use simple words that are readily recognized, such as *problem* rather than *glitch*, *break* rather than *fracture*.

Repeat. It helps to repeat what you have said using different words. When looking for a synonym, however, beware of cognates, words in other languages that look and sound similar to English words. The most common mistakes occur between English and Spanish. While *largo* in Spanish looks like *large*, it means *long;* and *embarazada* does not mean *embarrassed* but, rather, *pregnant*.

Expect confusion. It bears repeating that cultural influences that discourage giving a negative response will make it difficult for some people to say no. Do not ask whether someone understands and automatically take a yes to mean that he or she does. Instead of asking, watch for nonverbal signs of confusion in facial expressions or for behavior that shows you whether the person understands. Ask questions that require a choice among options rather than a yes or no response.

Get help. Whenever possible get the help of an interpreter, someone who is fluent enough in both languages to make things clear to all parties. Make sure, however, that the interpreter understands the concepts you are communicating. Following are guidelines for using interpreters and translators.

Getting Help in Interpreting

According to one physician, bilingual herself, patients prefer providers who understand them directly and they seek out those who speak their language fluently. That is not always feasible, however. Utilizing the help of interpreters, though essentially a stopgap measure, can go a long way in communicating across language barriers. Hospitals and clinics have found a number of ways to obtain and access such help.

Use a rotating interpreter bank. At one hospital, all staff who speak other languages are listed by language on a master list. When an interpreter is needed, the next person on the list is called so that no one individual is overburdened. One of the most frequent complaints of bilingual staff, however, is that this extra duty takes time away from their regular work and leaves them continuously backed up. Another occasional complaint is that they have been asked to interpret when the health care professional does not want to give bad news, such as telling the family that a loved one has died in the emergency room.

Hire a full-time interpreter. Many hospitals with a large non-English-speaking clientele employ full-time interpreters who are on call twenty-four hours a day. These professionally trained interpreters understand the culture and language of the patient and the medical information in the messages being sent. One hospital with a 70 percent Latino patient base trains its own interpreters by recruiting unemployed individuals in its community who are receiving Aid to Families with Dependent Children (AFDC) and putting them through an intensive training program. Although they generally are already conversationally bilingual, they are given training in hospital procedure, medical terminology, and professionalism. Once trained, they "intern" in various units in the hospital before they are officially hired, often by the unit where they interned. Their assistance means extended service to the largely Latino population served by the hospital, and bilingual help for staff on each unit.

Pay for bilingual skills. Many organizations give an additional pay increment for staff who have and use bilingual skills on the job. Managers often are required to document the need for the use of the second language. In other cases employees applying for the bilingual pay differential are required to pass written and oral proficiency tests in the second language in order to be certified.

Hire or train bilingual staff. Bilingual proficiency is more frequently becoming a job requirement in hiring staff. In addition, second language training is offered in many health care organizations to help staff communicate with patients and coworkers from both sides of the language divide. English and Spanish tend to be the most frequently taught languages.

Utilize a language hot line. AT&T provides a twenty-four-hour language hot line to which many hospitals subscribe. The service provides on-call interpreters in most of the world's languages who can be accessed with a phone call. This service can be especially helpful when dealing with a less common language.

Create an informal network. When the previous methods are unavailable, the informal method of calling a bilingual employee for help is probably the most common. This system can work if the employee called has a good command of both languages and an understanding of the information that needs to be communicated. Such spur-of-the-moment aides would probably be able to relay directions in their own departments. These impromptu interpreters would probably find it difficult, however, to explain a complicated medical procedure. Another caution regarding this method is the tendency for fellow expatriates to "normalize" a patient's description to prevent embarrassment to the interpreter or to the patient. The following incident was described in the *Journal of Nervous and Mental Disease:* "A hospital janitor fluent in Spanish was asked to help translate for a Cuban patient whom police had brought to the emergency room for bizarre behavior in public. Mental status and psychiatric interviewing were entirely negative. Another staff translator was called, who arrived to hear the janitor telling the patient, "Don't tell them that; they'll think you're crazy." Subsequent evaluation with the second translator revealed the presence of delusions and command hallucinations."[7]

Use family members. In health care settings it is even more probable that family members will be used. Children, because they tend to learn English quicker than their parents, are often called upon. While use of family members may seem convenient, it brings its own set of problems. Patients may be reticent to disclose personal information in front of relatives. In the case of children, respect for their elders may make it awkward if not impossible for them to ask certain questions of their parents, grandparents, aunts, or uncles.

Guidelines for Using Interpreters

The following list offers guidelines for increasing effectiveness in communicating with the help of an interpreter.[8]

1. *Use a professionally trained interpreter whenever possible.* The individual should be fluent in both languages, trained in conveying meaning, not just translating vocabulary, and knowledgeable about medical procedures.

2. *When possible, use an interpreter who is older than the patient.* People of most other cultures have respect for older individuals and this may aid the process.

3. *When possible, use an interpreter of the same sex.* This makes communication about sensitive personal matters more comfortable.

4. *When possible, choose an interpreter from a similar sociopolitical background as the patient.* This avoids any ethnic or political rivalries that may hinder communication.

5. *Introduce the interpreter formally at the beginning of the conversation.* This shows respect to all concerned.

6. *Address the patient, not the interpreter.* Continue to face the patient, observing nonverbal behavior and making eye contact without staring.

7. *When possible, meet with the interpreter ahead of time.* Explain the case and your objectives in the session.

8. *Speak clearly, simply, and slowly.* Use simple sentences and words, and pause, giving the interpreter time to relay information. Allow time for extended conversations between interpreter and patient. Avoid complicated medical terminology. However, maintain a professional manner and do not talk down to the patient. Encourage questions or corrections from the interpreter and patient.

Avoiding Mishaps in Translation

Bilingual and multilingual communication is commonly seen in hospitals across the country because nonnative English speakers make up a significant percentage of the population in many metropolitan areas. In attempting to reach these populations, however, some organizations miss the boat by providing poorly translated material. In one case, a hospital attempting to reach its limited-English-speaking staff had its newsletter printed bilingually. The Spanish portion was so poorly written, however, with grammatical and spelling errors, that the Spanish-speaking staff were insulted. Monica Moreno, intercultural communication expert and certified translator, offers the following advice to ensure accurate, appropriate translations that achieve the desired communication objective:[9]

1. *The translator should be a native speaker of the language in which he or she is writing.* Although Monica, a native of Argentina, is fluent in English, Italian, and French, she writes only Spanish translations, because that is her native tongue.

2. *A translation should be edited by a native speaker from a different country than the translator's.* Monica, for example, might have a native of Cuba or Mexico edit her translation. This is especially important in the Spanish-speaking world, where regional and national differences in vocabulary and expressions can cause confusion. Puerto Rican Spanish may be very different from Nicaraguan, Peruvian, or Chilean Spanish.

3. *Use a professional translator.* This expertise is certified in many other countries; in the United States, however, it is not. Therefore, checking the translator's references and having a native speaker read samples of the translator's work can be used to verify skill levels. A professional understands the nuances of communication and has the ability to adjust the translation to suit the target group.

4. *Augment the written translation with a question and answer session.* If the document relates to policies and procedures, there are apt to be questions. Holding a session in the employees' native language in which they can get clarification, verify their understanding, and discuss implications can be helpful in ensuring that the information is understood.

5. *Budget for translation.* This is a prime example of the saying, "If it's worth doing, it's worth doing right." Having an important message written by an executive, checked by the legal department, reviewed by human resources, and translated by an employee who does not have the requisite education is asking for trouble. Include the cost of translation in the budget for any program that needs to be communicated to non-English-speaking employees or patients.

6. *If you use bilingual staff to translate, verify the translation.* Check for accuracy by having another bilingual employee translate the document back into English.

7. *Provide the option of translation in a nondiscriminatory way.* If you ask patients or staff if they want a translation of a document, they are apt to say no because they do not want to be a burden or expose their lack of English skills. It is more effective to offer the option in a matter-of-fact way, providing stacks of handouts or brochures, with each stack in a different language.

Culturally Sensitive Medical Interviews

Medical interviews are often difficult even when all parties speak the same language and come from similar backgrounds. The discomfort or pain as well as worry and fear coupled with the sensitive and intimate nature of the information needed often make for an awkward, uncomfortable interaction. When language and cultural differences are added to the equation, the obstacles increase. Not only is there danger of misunderstanding, but unintentional cultural blunders may block communication and create wrong impressions on both sides of the interchange.

As uncomfortable or unpleasant as it is anticipated to be, most patients of any background expect to have an examination. Beyond this initial understanding, however, expectations diverge. According to Katalanos, most Southeast Asian patients have not had experience giving a standard Western medical history and do not recognize Western disease classifications, so a typical review of systems process would be confusing. In addition, Southeast Asian patients generally desire an explanation of their illness after only a few questions. An immediate diagnosis raises the esteem of the doctor in the eyes of the patient and increases confidence in his or her ability.[10] This expectation might seem unrealistic to a Western provider, whose interpretation of the diagnostic process is more complex, but in Southeast Asia general or vague statements are acceptable. "I can see you are having trouble with your heart" is an acceptable explanation at this stage.

Let us take a look at the stages in the medical interview process and consider what adaptations or modifications might be called for to get the most complete and accurate information and to build rapport and a trusting relationship between patient and health care professional.

Preparation

In preparing for the interview it is important to find out as much as possible about the patient beforehand so you can have the necessary resources available. What is the patient's language capability, including native language, proficiency in English, and/or any other language he or she speaks that you also speak? Make arrangements for an interpreter if one will be needed. Have literature available in the patient's language if appropriate. Also investigate the patient's cultural background. If you are unfamiliar with the norms and values of this culture, get information from colleagues, from other cultural informants, or from books or articles.

Introductions

The beginning of your encounter is a critical stage in setting the tone and creating initial impressions. Address the patient, or if he or she is in a group, address the eldest male first, giving your formal name and title and using whatever title (Mr., Mrs., Miss, Professor) is appropriate to address the other person. Other than shaking hands, it is wise to avoid touching, such as guiding the person by touching his or her back or by putting your hand on his or her shoulder, because this may be perceived as insulting or demeaning.

Explain the need for the information you will be requesting as well as the parts of the exam. For example, you might say, "I'm going to ask you a few questions first, then I will need to have you lie on the table so I can do a physical examination." One female Cambodian woman, now a medical interpreter, reported an incident she experienced soon after her arrival in the United States. "When I first came to this country, I went to the doctor and was told to take off my clothes. I was scared and did not know the reason for this. I had an eight-year-old to interpret because I did not speak English. I would not do it, and I left the clinic because I did not understand and was embarrassed."[11]

The Interview

In conducting the interview, ask questions as simply as possible, avoiding compound sentences and clinical terminology. "Have you ever had trouble with your heart beating too fast?" is much more understandable than "Have you ever had episodes of palpitations?" In addition to investigating the immediate condition and symptoms, you will need to find out the history of the problem, the patient's perception of the cause, and any treatment that has been attempted. "Were you ever ill with this before?" "What do you think is the cause?" "What have you done about this?" and "Have you taken any medicines or gone to a doctor or healer before?" would be appropriate questions.

The Family Practice Residency at San Jose Health Center in San Jose, California, offers the following LEARN guidelines for overcoming obstacles in cross-cultural communication with patients:[12]

L	Listen with sympathy and understanding of the patient's perception of the problem.
E	Explain your perceptions of the problem.
A	Acknowledge and discuss the differences and similarities.
R	Recommend treatment.
N	Negotiate agreement.

Listen. The object of this first step is to draw out the patient's thoughts about his or her condition, its cause, and the preferred treatment. Berlin and Fowkes suggest questions such as, "What do you feel may be causing your problem?" "How do you feel this illness is affecting you?" and "What do you feel might be of benefit?"[13]

Tripp-Reimer, Brink, and Saunders suggest additional questions, including "Why do you think it started when it did?" "How severe is your sickness? Will it have a long or short duration?" and "What do you fear about your sickness?"[14]

Explain. Helping the patient understand the Western biomedical model is the focus at this stage. This model may be different from the patient's conception; it is important, however, that he or she understand the caregiver's reason and strategy.

Acknowledge. At this stage it is important for the caregiver to acknowledge the patient's explanation and find some agreement between it and that of the provider, if possible. If it is not possible, then there is still the need to acknowledge understanding of the patient's explanation and to use it to find a different way to help the patient grasp the provider's view. For example, if the patient believes that blood is irreplaceable and that loss of it causes weakness, the physician could explain the quantity of blood in the body, the amount that can safely be removed, and the time it takes for regeneration by the body.

Recommend. At this point, the caregiver proposes a treatment plan with the patient's involvement. Understanding the patient's lifestyle and preferences is important so that the plan will be followed. For example, rather than telling a patient who does not eat dairy products to take medication with milk, asking the patient what beverages he or she drinks and choosing the most appropriate one might be helpful. Finding out when the patient takes meals, then recommending that medications or procedures be done in conjunction with them ("Take one with breakfast and one with dinner") might be more effective than giving time-related prescriptions such as "Soak your wrist every four hours during the day."

Negotiate. Finally, ask the patient how the plan would work and be willing to modify it. If the patient does not eat breakfast and the medication needs to be taken with food, negotiate with the patient something that would be palatable for him or her to eat, or find a different schedule for the medication. If the patient does not want to go through chemotherapy because of the burden it would put on loved ones, you might suggest that not stopping the spread of the disease and not prolonging life would be a much greater burden on them.

The patient's buy-in, which is developed throughout the LEARN steps, is essential to successful treatment and recovery. Although this process may take more time initially, it pays off in the long run. As Cher Vang, a Hmong parent representative at St. Paul Children's Hospital stated, "If they [Western doctors] spend a little more time and build trust, in the long run I think we can get things done easier. If the Hmong people trust you, then they will allow you to do whatever you want to do, because they know you aren't going to do any harm."[15]

Communication is essential to healing. The wider your repertoire of methods and approaches to sending and receiving information, and to creating understanding and building relationships with patients and coworkers, the greater will be your effectiveness.

6

Removing Stereotypes
That Block High-Quality Care

The word *stereotype* can be defined as "a fixed image." Although stereotypes can be positive images of people, places, or things, most often they have negative connotations that influence the dynamics of interpersonal interactions and the opportunities or obstacles we experience in life. This chapter explores how these fixed images become harmful or limiting to both health care providers and health care receivers. Employees, patients, and families lose when we perpetuate stereotypes. Sometimes the generalizations are benign, but the cumulative effect of a repeated image, accurate or not, takes its toll over time. Just look at the following stereotypical thoughts and consider what their impacts might be:

- Foreign-trained physicians receive substandard education and give lower-quality care.
- Doctors care more about making money than they do about the well-being of their patients.
- Surgeons are elitist prima donnas.
- Immigrants take advantage of health care services.
- Nurses are altruistic nurturers.
- Women make good general practitioners, but they are not cut out to be surgeons.

What makes these or other such images stereotypes is that over time they have come to be commonly held perceptions. While there may be some altruistic nurses, some bigoted whites, or some immigrants who abuse health care services, not all nurses are altruistic, not all whites are bigoted, and not all immigrants overuse or abuse the health care system. But health-care-specific stereotypes as well as more general ones can shape interactions in a health care environment. A patient who perceives that whites are bigots may not trust the white admitting clerk and hold back important information. A manager who perceives that blacks always feel like victims might buy into that victim mentality and shortchange black employees by unconsciously withholding helpful feedback that could enhance their professional growth. An administrator who buys into the assumption that Asians have exceptional quantitative skills may, when it comes to hiring or promoting people for jobs with a strong need for interpersonal skills, discount, or avoid considering altogether, any talented Asians for managerial positions.

The sad fact is that holding preconceived and categorical views, however erroneous they are, is a common human response designed to increase safety in a complex world. Although these generalizations may occasionally serve a useful purpose, more often they limit our perceptions about individuals and about their capabilities. The problem with stereotypes is that when we meet individuals who challenge them, we exceptionalize those individuals. In other words, we look at them as being different. What we do not seem to do is question the stereotype itself; but we need to.

The Realities of Stereotypes

To manage stereotypes effectively, that is, to minimize them and their negative impact, some basic realities need to be understood.

Stereotypes are part of the human condition. It is not possible to be human and avoid involvement with stereotypes, either as victim or perpetrator. The danger comes when one becomes unable to move beyond the limits of one's stereotypes. For example, in many health care facilities throughout California, Florida, the Southwest, and New York, the housekeeping staff is often composed of primarily Hispanic employees, many of whom are new immigrants and speak little or no English. A possible, dangerous stereotype here would be that because of effective job performance by these employees, all Hispanics would be slated for housekeeping and none for accounting, the business office, or management.

Stereotypes are accumulated by osmosis. They are like secondhand smoke; you do not need a direct hit to be negatively affected. The fixed images of print and visual media serve up a relentless number of mental pictures. For example, in the health care field, the belief exists that high-priced physicians provide higher quality medical treatment than those who treat the poor. Although there may be cases where this is true, higher cost does not always equate to higher quality. The assumptions either way have a downside for the patient as consumer. On the one hand, if a person pays a lot of money for care, he may have a misplaced and total faith in a physician and not ask enough pertinent questions. On the other hand, there are many excellent doctors who practice medicine at understaffed and overcrowded county hospitals that serve low-income patients.

Another example of stereotype busting involves a business man who went through treatment for lymphoma. At the outset, he had far more faith in his U.S.-born-and-trained physician than he had in a foreign-born doctor who also treated him. Over time, however, he came to feel very differently and eventually would not go back to the original U.S.-born physician, who had treated him previously for other diagnoses. Through repeated personal experience and because of his open mind, his stereotype no longer existed.

We are all both victims and perpetrators of stereotypes. Part of being human means labeling other people, but when we do this we put them in a box and perpetuate stereotypes. Other people put us in those same boxes, and when it happens it feels belittling. While we are busy classifying others in some fixed category, the same is being done to us. Though other groups consider whites racist more frequently than they consider other groups racist, there is certainly ample evidence to show that whites can also be the targets of prejudice. For example, the authors, two white females who teach diversity seminars, have had several people of color consider not attending our sessions. They signed up not knowing our skin color, but when they first saw us they assumed there was little that two white people could teach them about diversity. Their view was that we could not possibly understand their reality or have something meaningful to offer them because as whites we have had immense privilege in our society and have faced few of the obstacles they have, such as institutionalized racism. Although it is true that a white person cannot know what it is like to be black, for example, it is not true that the universal parts of our human experience do not enable us to connect with or learn from one another. These particular participants were elated that they chose to stay and attend our session, not only because of significant subject matter gains but especially because their most basic assumptions about race, privilege, and being human were challenged. The truth is that lighter skin or being female or any other fact of life has both advantages and disadvantages. But the point here is that seminar participants who had no experience of our work but lots of experience with other whites almost did not give us a chance. Fortunately, they did. They learned much and were glad they stayed.

The issue for health care practitioners is to come to terms with the stereotypes they hold based on a variety of factors, such as socioeconomics, race, education, gender, and so many others. Look at your underlying assumptions about the socioeconomic, ethnic, religious, or racial groups you serve. Though it may be human to hold stereotypes, it is very important to recognize them so they do not control you and your interactions with other employees or with patients and their families. You can enhance your ability to manage this process by using yourself as a case in point. Think about what it means to be the victim of stereotypes and see how your own opportunities are enhanced or diminished. Figure 6.1 is useful as an example of limitations you might face as a white female, a physician over age fifty, or the chief financial officer of your organization. These three examples are designed to illustrate how you can apply the Figure 6.2 worksheet to your own reality.

Once you have identified cases where you are the object of others' stereotypes, spend some time discussing the following questions with a colleague or two:

1. How does it feel to consider how others might perceive you?

Figure 6.1 Stereotype Examples.

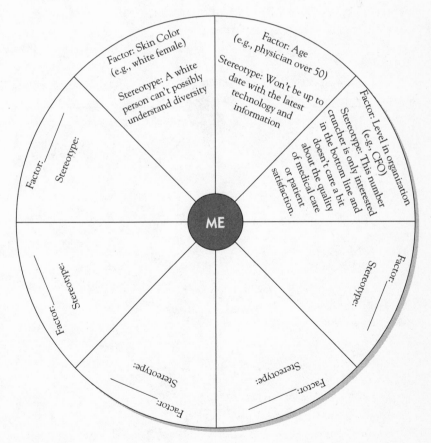

Figure 6.2 You as the Object of Stereotypes.

Directions: In each of the spaces below, identify factors on which others may stereotype you. The areas for stereotyping are vast and can range from field of work or level within the organization to skin color, gender, age, marital status, or geographic region. Then jot down the stereotypical assumptions held about you because of that factor. The point of this exercise is to see where you might be limited by others' perceptions about you.

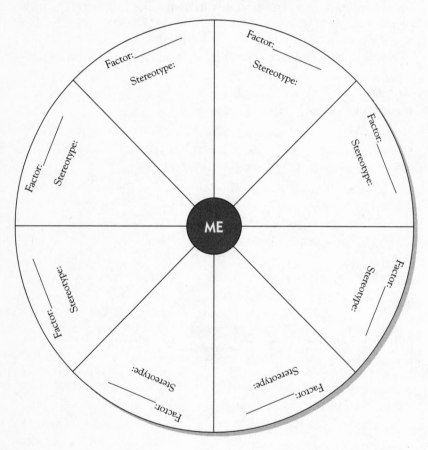

2. Where do you feel misunderstood and/or limited by others?

3. What reaction does their perception (or misperception) bring out in you, and what if anything can you do about it?

4. How might their views about you affect your career opportunities, your interactions with people throughout the organization, or your relationships with patients?

5. When do you make the same misjudgments about other people?

6. What does the habitual, but unconscious, reliance or stereotype mean as you try to create an organization in which all employees reach their full potential?

Stereotypes are self-fulfilling prophecies. The *Los Angeles Times* cited a recent study by Stanford University's Claude Steele, which suggests that poor performance by blacks and others is linked to a fear of fulfilling negative images.[1] Steele, a social psychologist, studied differences in performance between blacks and whites. The expected culprits, such as social class, genetics, lack of academic skills, dysfunctional families, or living in a segregated society, are not guilty. Steele's theory is that blacks, or members of any group bombarded with and made anxious by negative stereotypes, wonder about the truth of these stereotypes. He refers to this condition of anxiety, of being judged by a negative stereotype, as *stereotype threat*. When men are told often enough that they are insensitive and unfeeling, or the elderly are told often enough that they are slow and limited, the perception and burden it brings actually hinders performance.

Steele's theory has been lab tested on campus at Stanford University. Steele and colleague Joshua Aronson of the University of Texas suggest that this stereotype anxiety can be applied to any group, not just to blacks. In fact, they note that the scores of white males on tests that measure quantitative skills plummeted when told they would be measured against Asians. Steele's most meaningful work regarding stereotype threat has involved experiments to raise the performance of black students and reduce the black college student dropout rate from a high of 70 percent. His theory is applicable to other groups. If you apply the principal of stereotype threat to your hospital staff, where does anxiety about the negative perceptions of others exist in your organization? What is the impact of this negative self-perception on the performance of people in certain job classifications, ethnic groups, or geographic regions? How do these negative images affect people's willingness to take risks, try for advancement, or attain promotion?

Anxiety due to others' negative perceptions also affects customer service. For example, do patients and their families enter your facilities with negative expectations? If so, on what are these perceptions based? How might these views influence their experience? When might you lose patients because negative perceptions exist about safety? About the quality of care? About the attentiveness of staff? About the ability to have staff who speak the patient's language? Health care environments intimidate and produce anxiety under the best of circumstances, but if you add to that equation how people perceive they might be treated or cared for as a member of a certain group, you can see the potential for a less than satisfactory experience.

The Realities of Human Nature

The realities of stereotyping just discussed are impossible to eliminate. The best we can do is be aware of our own blind spots and assumptions, and challenge ourselves not to fall prey to the fixed images that continue floating around the environment. Monitoring ourselves is almost a full-time job, but once we see how pervasive stereotypes are and how much a part of being human they are, we can then manage our own biases and assumptions more effectively. The process will, however, necessitate understanding the realities of human nature as well as the realities of stereotypes.

Like attracts like. Opposites may attract in romance novels, but in real life people generally gravitate toward those who are like them. The predictability of behavior and the similarities shared in common engender trust, which increases comfort. For example, a cartoon in a recent issue of a business magazine shows two identical men sitting across the desk from one another at a hiring interview. The hiring official says, "You're just the kind of person I've been looking for." Like this cartoon character, most of us tend to prefer people who mirror us, if not in appearance then in values, lifestyle, and behavior.

People are unaware of their biases. Biases and preferences are usually unconscious, and are formed from the powerful secondhand smoke that is in the environment. The values and beliefs that shape our decisions are deep in our unconscious. We believe that we are acting from free will and independent thinking when in fact some subtle programming is at work.

Studies have focused on the frequency with which teachers call on male students in proportion to how often they call on female students. Males are called on much more frequently. When well-meaning teachers are shown the discrepancy, they are not only horrified but surprised at their complete lack of awareness of this tendency. If a teacher inadvertently acknowledges boys over twelve years of age more than girls, what might the cumulative effect be? In a work context, we may give more help to one employee than to another. Perhaps we give a more detailed explanation or spend more time exploring treatment options when we feel more comfortable with one patient than we do with another.

Recognizing prejudice is painful and threatening. Examining our own biases is an uncomfortable and often painful process. When faced with proof that we do hold preconceived notions, we often feel attacked and respond defensively, giving rational arguments for our irrational views. When we spend our energy arguing back and defending ourselves, we do not examine our behavior and views. We get locked into old patterns, entrenched responses, and knee-jerk reactions that we are reluctant to question.

Managing Your Biases:
Suggestions for Fighting Stereotypes

We have discussed how deep and unconscious stereotypes can be. The important next step is to challenge our assumptions about people as a way to manage our biases. Not all assumptions are negative, but even positive expectations can hurt. Any generalization is limiting because it prevents us from understanding the real individual before us. Also, positive expectations predispose us to give better treatment to some patients or coworkers, and less attention or help to others.

The most important questions about stereotypes and prejudice in health care revolve around their impact on the quality of care offered to patients and the productivity of the workforce. You need to consider where assumptions and stereotypes are limiting opportunities to serve people effectively. You can also explore whether stereotypes are inhibiting your ability to attract a broader patient base: Do you have good word of mouth in the community?

Beyond becoming aware, you can take the following concrete steps to address limiting assumptions: question your assumptions, question others' assumptions, break down barriers, chip away at your discomfort with differences, and be honest with yourself. In fact, now is a good time to try doing these very things.

Question your assumptions. Keep yourself in check by listening to your own attitudes and by asking yourself hard questions. Start with paying very close attention to language, particularly to your use of *them* and *they*. This is usually a sign of unconsciously grouping people. Are "they" really that different from you? The phrase "those people" is a clear giveaway that assumptions are about to follow. Keep looking for common ground rather than differences. Try to develop empathy and an appreciation for similar experiences by remembering times when you have felt like acting or have acted in some of the ways you are seeing others act. Such attention helps you to focus on shared interests and common humanity.

Pay attention to your subtle preferences. If you meet a roomful of strangers, ask yourself why you chose to talk to a particular person. On the job, try to notice any patterns you have with patients or coworkers—those to whom you are drawn and whom you tolerate, and those you tend to discount. What assumptions underlie all these choices? With both patients and coworkers, the patterns will be telling.

Once you get into the habit of checking your assumptions you will pay more attention to how they get formulated. When there is a void, human beings metaphorically become writers who busily assign motive, values, and beliefs to others. These assumptions may be reinforced by images from the nightly news, a recent movie, or today's newspaper. Such media influence is often insidious. For example, the book *Don't Believe the Hype*, by Farai Chedya, reported an analysis of sports news coverage for National Football League and National Collegiate Athletic Association games in 1988–89. Fully 75 percent of the adjectives used to describe white football players referred to brains, while 65 percent of those used for black players referred to brawn. In basketball, 63 percent of comments referred to white players' brains, and 77 percent referred to black players' brawn. Finally, 80 percent of references to stupid plays were about blacks.[2]

Assumptions may also arise from previous experience with similar situations. If the admitting department, for example, has had repeated experience with limited English speakers, its expectations may turn out to be accurate, or they may still be way off base. The first step is to recognize such assumptions and take them for what they are—estimates and guesses rather than reality. Then you can question your assumptions, consider alternate views, and investigate to achieve more accurate predictions or assessments. Once you get into the habit of analyzing what you see and hear, fixed expectations will cease to be so influential in your choices.

Awareness begins at home. What are the messages you tell yourself when you see patient or family behaviors? What other assumptions might be possible? Having a sense of your own button pushers can help you get past the conditioned response. Each person who has contact with a patient can influence that patient's perception of the health care experience, and so many of the factors that help us size a person up are subtle. Bringing awareness to usually unconscious responses will undoubtedly result in better care for all patients.

Question others' assumptions. Though assumptions are pervasive and potentially harmful, they can be challenged and their negative effects minimized. When you think of or hear a negative comment or erroneous assumption, counter it with an example that refutes the view. You might also ask the individual to give examples that support their view, and do so in a tone that is hospitable as opposed to belligerent or argumentative. "When was the last time that happened to you?" is a question you can ask in a nonthreatening way. When someone complains about that dirty homeless person who has lice, you can say, "A child in my own daughter's classroom had lice. It's not an affliction of only the dirty or the homeless."

Break down barriers. The most positive, favorable cross-cultural encounters seem to involve food and breaking bread together. Make it a point to once a week talk with, sit by, or have lunch with someone you do not know well. It might be a coworker from another culture, a colleague with a different educational background, or someone from another generation. Spend time in the community your hospital serves. If you can do so, make time to have lunch at local restaurants or patronize other businesses in the neighborhood. The more diverse the cuisine, the better. In the process of sharing and relationship building, you will get to know people as individuals, not as statistical categories.

Chip away at discomfort with differences. Increasing your comfort level with differences comes only with practice. Just as a new pair of shoes can pinch when you wear them for the first time, a new behavior may feel a little uncomfortable initially. However, the shoes do not get broken in by staying in a box in the closet, and neither do the new behaviors become second nature unless you use them. Put yourself in situations where you are with people who are different from you. Look for things you may have in common with colleagues or with patients and their families who come from other backgrounds. Challenge your predictable and all too human preference for the familiar, and congratulate yourself for living through the twinges of discomfort at the beginning of new and different experiences.

Be honest with yourself. Making generalizations about people and categorizing them into groups does not mean that you are a bigot. It just means you are human. It may also mean that you have repeated an experience enough times to generalize from it. It is only when you admit your own assumptions, however, and the fact that generalizations sometimes become fixed images (that is, stereotypes), that you can keep them from directing your behavior and causing you to misjudge others. Be honest about your own reactions to different patient norms and behaviors, or to various obstacles to delivering competent care. The challenge is to look at the patient in front of you and notice the mental tapes you might be playing. Use the information and awareness about stereotypes to alter the messages you give yourself.

The point of this chapter has not been to finger-point, blame, or label anyone as racist or bigoted. Rather it has been designed to demonstrate the universal phenomenon of labeling and stereotyping people and ultimately limiting their performance, opportunity, behavior, and commitment. Although there is no way to eradicate stereotypes and assumptions from human experience, awareness, insight, and information can soften their blow and make the deleterious effects less so. Following this path is a lifetime job and requires tenacity and commitment, but it is a job worth doing!

7

The Diversity Leadership Challenge

It is difficult not to wonder why some organizations attain greatness and navigate tumultuous transitions effectively while others with similar resources and strengths do not. Studies reveal that organizations that achieve results and maintain high performance have the necessary leadership. The gap between an organization's future vision and its current reality is narrowed with the help of excellent leadership. Realizing the benefits of long-term cultural change takes a leader of great vision, conviction, courage, and patience. The adventure can be precarious because the word *diversity* is loaded and often pushes buttons, derailing potentially fruitful transitions. In this challenging climate the exploration of leadership and change is not only legitimate but essential.

For our purposes in this chapter, the leadership concept includes not only the positional power of CEOs and other high-level administrators, but also leaders at any level—situational leaders who can influence the behavior of others.

The Essentials of Diversity Leadership

An astute leader understands the strategic thinking that is necessary to outmaneuver the competition and win the hearts and minds of his or her own staff. But also important is the ability to make the intangible concrete. Here are ten essential characteristics that we have observed in successful leaders of health care diversity efforts.

Be Driven by Meaning

A recent article on leadership in *Fortune* magazine quotes the *I Ching,* a Chinese leadership guide used by Confucius: "Radical changes require adequate authority. A man must have inner strength as well as influential position. What he does must correspond with a higher truth. . . . If a revolution is not founded on such inner truth, the results are bad and it has no success. For in the end, men will support only those undertakings which they feel instinctively to be just."[1]

Sisters of Providence Health Systems (SPHS), headquartered in Seattle but operating in Alaska, the Pacific Northwest, and Southern California's San Fernando Valley, clearly illustrates the importance of having a sense of inner truth and justice. This system is being led in its diversity effort by Sister Karen Dufault. She has inherited an organization whose values permeate all aspects of the work it does and the decisions it makes about how to deliver care and allocate resources. Respect, justice, compassion, and excellence are front and center during discussions about how to deliver care and serve those who cannot pay, or who may be gay and HIV positive in a Catholic hospital.

Sister Karen's leadership is essential to ensuring that everyone who has an encounter at SPHS, whether employee or patient, sees the organization's mission and values lived out, and that patients sense that all staff members are contributing their very best to the service of others. She does this by staying in close touch with each of the service areas and by holding all SPHS employees accountable for sensitive and compassionate care. By being visible in a video distributed throughout this large system in which she discusses the importance of diversity at every level of the organization, and by visiting service areas, her passion and commitment to serving all people within SPHS in a sensitive and compassionate way is clear. In tight economic times, when resources are scarce for all health care institutions, SPHS reaches out and strives for the opportunity to serve a population that at times presents linguistic, ethnic, geographic, and financial challenges. Sister Karen's meaning-driven leadership helps large numbers of people both internal and external to the system.[2]

Take the Long View

Long-term change is a hard sell in American culture. Executive wisdom and leadership always necessitate juggling priorities and knowing when to change those priorities on the basis of signals from the macroclimate. Maintaining commitment on tough issues that are perceived to be important builds trust and credibility and avoids the tempting "program du jour" mentality that infects so many hospitals and health care facilities.

Mark Meyers, current CEO of West Hills Hospital in the San Fernando Valley and former CEO of Coastal Communities Hospital in Santa Ana, California, has spent his adult life in health care leadership and management. He is a strategic thinker willing to let the results be demonstrated long term. An example of his long-range view involves his participation in California's health care system twenty years ago. The population involved were the immigrant poor in hospitals concentrated primarily in Orange County. Among this group it was common practice to come to emergency rooms or to gynecologists for the first time right before delivery. As a whole, this population had no experience with prenatal care. The consequence was increased costs to the state for babies born with numerous health problems. Under the leadership of Meyers and others, Medi-Cal invested in educating this population about prenatal care. Today, twenty years later, with no more Medi-Cal for immigrants and with health care benefits severely cut, this patient population continues to opt for prenatal care, often paying for it themselves.

Here is a long-term investment in training and education for the betterment of all parties involved.[3]

Demonstrate Commitment Through Investing Resources

Because talk is cheap, it has been exhilarating to find examples of leaders who steer their organization toward putting its money where its mouth is.

One such example we relish close to our own community involves St. Francis Hospital in Lynwood, California. This Catholic hospital, located in a working class community, has stated that part of its mission is to serve the poor. This hospital reaches into the community to identify young people who are underskilled and unemployed and trains them to become nurse aides and licensed vocational nurses. The program has provoked occasional concern from nurses because some of the new employees do not meet the very high standards of performance the nurses would like. But the hospital remains committed to putting its resources back into its community. The investment so far has benefited the larger community, which gains a more skilled workforce, individuals who now have jobs (many for the first time), and an institution that is building relationships with the community it serves. The hospital is seen as an extremely helpful force. Some of the newly employed feel a profound new dignity and sense of belonging.[4]

Base Decisions on the Core Values of the Organization

Being true to the values of the organization is the leadership quality that often pits organizational financial health against personal integrity. In the ideal world, those two values support and reinforce rather than conflict with one another. In a cost-conscious health care climate, however, economic incentives take on the aura of Big Brother. Executives want their institutions to be economically viable, to promote health, and to be accessible to the community.

Most leaders we interviewed work hard to do all three, but they understand the rarity of that occurrence, and therein lies the challenge.

Yotaro Kobayashi, chairman of Fuji Xerox and successor to Akio Morita as Japan's best-known international industrialist, was quoted on a topic relevant to leadership, core values, and diversity. He said, "As our activities become global, understanding the people in different parts of the world—all the way to the roots of their thinking—is very important. That means understanding the factors on which their values and sense of judgment are based."[5] Although Kobayashi was referring to Fuji Xerox's global consumer base, health care institutions in many regions of the United States are also global entities. Understanding the values of patients, all the way to the roots of their thinking, is essential. For many of you, the world not only is at your door, it has entered your house. Excellent leadership sends the message that there is no time like the present to begin appreciating and understanding these values as you welcome your guests.

Engage in Creative, Open-Minded Thinking

Excellent leadership involves expanding individual and collective problem-solving capabilities. This is done through a climate of innovation that welcomes trying new things, encourages sharing new ideas even if they are still in the developmental stages, and reinforces exploring unproven strategies. Although the risks in an open climate may be a bit higher, so are the rewards.

Creativity is especially critical when dealing with diversity-related issues because the dilemmas are complex, and although conventional answers are being considered, few solutions have proven to be universal. What is needed is a sense of *ethnorelativity*. This is the recognition that good ideas and solutions come from a variety of places. The two-way street metaphor of cultural sensitivity on one side and acculturation on the other presumes that all parties have a piece of truth, and that when you mix all of them together you not only get more avenues for pursuing successful accomplishment of goals but you also remake the culture in the process. Openness and creativity become the primary modus operandi rather than behavior that advertises "This is how we've always done it here."

For a leader who desires an open culture, the next step beyond the two-way street metaphor is to shed some of the ethnocentrism that is part of the human condition. We all see the world through our own eyes and experiences; our way is the right way. Executive leaders who are ethnorelative—who believe that appropriateness is not necessarily measured by one's own standard but rather by any number of standards that have different viewpoints and definitions of appropriateness—demonstrate that there are at least several ways to skin the proverbial cat, and in so doing they role-model leader behavior that fosters a creative climate. An ethnorelative mentality assumes that all ideas add value and offer something for consideration, while presuming that no one idea is intrinsically superior. Leaders who promote this open-minded thinking can perhaps shape this same mind-set among staff and patients.

Finally, in shaping this open environment, the leader, manager, or supervisor will probably have both creativity and conflict. These two elements are a natural part of the creative process that can lead to real gains from diversity. Sometimes you even experience creativity and conflict simultaneously. The end results should be enhanced openness in thinking and an expanded view of how to define and solve problems cross-culturally so that more effective solutions are ultimately produced.

This sort of open-minded thinking can be role-modeled and demonstrated at any level of the organization. The authors remember when an administrator capitalized on the help of a very sharp security guard at Children's Hospital of Los Angeles who demonstrated an adaptable way of thinking and problem solving. He also demonstrated necessary cultural competence, so this story is a twofer. Here is what happened.

One night during evening visiting hours, approximately twenty-five members of the Gypsy community, primary and extended family, came to visit one of their children. Because the child shared a room and because hospital policy mandates no more than two family members per patient at a time, the nurse tried to get all but two of the Gypsies to leave. They would not cooperate because they believed their presence was critical to the patient's emotional and physical healing. The charge nurse on duty that night went from patience to frustration to anger fairly quickly and called an administrator, who promptly called security. When security came and the administrator explained the situation to the guard, he said he knew a little something about Gypsy culture and he would like to handle the situation. He began by finding the oldest male in the group and then formally introduced both himself and the administrator, with name and title, to the leader of the clan. Once he made these formal introductions, a very appropriate practice in this hierarchical culture, he explained that hospital policy allowed two visitors per room. The security guard offered a nearby waiting room to the rest of the group and suggested rotating visitors, any two at a time. Case closed, problem solved. The combination of being culturally sensitive and knowing the values of the culture (hierarchical structure, status in gender and age, and welfare of the child paramount) proved helpful. In addition, the guard helped the visiting family to acculturate to hospital norms. Being ethnorelative in understanding the Gypsy culture and using an open-minded solution avoided conflict and created understanding. What the security guard did at an operational level leaders can do at the highest levels of the organization. Opening people's minds and role-modeling the appreciation of multiple viewpoints is a clear benefit for any organization.

Demand Accountability for Results but Offer Flexibility in Accomplishment

Enlightened leaders know what they want from their people and hold them accountable for doing the job. The corollary to that expectation is that if employees do not get results, there are consequences. Stratford Sherman says, "Insistence on accountability gives backbone to the softer stuff. All the model companies routinely fire people who don't meet their tough standards."[6]

But great leaders offer room for individuality in how to meet these goals. They recognize that one style does not fit all. In a health care industry dependent on science and technology for quality care, this flexibility and lack of a "right" way to do things is sometimes countercultural to the rigorous scientific climate that serves as a backdrop.

The ability to simultaneously maintain accountability and flexibility is a tightrope act and one of the most difficult arts of leadership. We see SPHS wrestling with this issue currently as they roll out diversity systemwide. They are in the process of juggling these two dimensions very successfully, but not without concern about how to do it well. For SPHS, consistency and accountability come in having every service area from Alaska to Southern California form a diversity council charged with leading the diversity effort. The council gets two days of training. The curriculum involves not only education about the organization's philosophy and its paradigm regarding diversity, but also about the business case, about appropriate terminology in discussing concepts related to culture (both organizational and ethnic), and about stereotypes, expectations, and assumptions. One entire day of training for this diversity council in each service area is designed to have the group define its own mission and create a strategy for achieving long-term culture change. The objective of the change process is a diversity-friendly place for all people who work in or are served by facilities operated by the staff of SPHS.

The diversity content and training are the same regardless of location and are based on clear organizational mission and goals. However, the way each organization goes about accomplishing its goals or what each chooses to focus on may differ. Even the time lines are fluid within clearly set parameters. This is flexibility in action.

In addition to the two days of training and planning for the SPHS diversity councils, each service area has designated that an in-house staff go through five days of facilitator training so that the education is conducted for all staff throughout the system. This is an ambitious, well-designed process. We believe that the flexibility that enables each service area to go its own way while still being held accountable for a result at the end of the process is appropriate. It is an excellent model for walking that very difficult tightrope. Accountability and flexibility can be a very powerful duo when properly used and balanced.[7]

Be Willing to Change, Grow, and Adapt

Leadership is now more than ever about leading the way through change. It involves explaining the context in which the carousel swirls. For example, one of the authors was a speaker several years ago at two conferences for the American College of Physician Executives. She conducted workshops on the role of the physician executive in leading physicians through the changes brought about by all the diversity having an impact on the health care industry. The seminar coincided with President Clinton's initial health reform proposal. Participants were not nearly as interested in exploring diversity as they were in discussing the health care revolution being suggested and debated at the national level. The buzz was about potential consequences, both fiscal and otherwise, of national policy. The sessions that looked at forming new health care partnerships were bursting with energy, anxiety, confusion, stimulation, and uncertainty. They drew far more people than those focused on operational issues. That was no surprise.

What was particularly eye-opening, however, was to see the question marks and concerns on the faces of people confronted with immense change, people who have always had some degree of control, status, dependable income, and power to influence the organization. They were now as worried about their fates and their futures as people we have met at lower levels of organizations where we have worked. The anxiety of change is magnified at lower levels of the organization, where control seems even less certain, status seems more questionable, income seems less dependable, and perceptions of power seem nonexistent. Leaders trying to create a motivating climate amid rapid change have their jobs cut out for them. It is difficult but necessary to try to minimize the anxiety so that employees can be functional rather than traumatized and paralyzed from worry about their futures. Although no leader can cushion the reality of impermanent jobs and a changing employer-employee relationship, how a leader role-models change and talks about it, keeps people informed, and listens does make a difference. Empathy can be a tremendous leadership asset. Those who are genuinely empathetic may have an edge in communicating honestly, respectfully, and with sensitivity. These skills can help employees move through change more easily.

The most effective health care leaders help employees to understand the fast and complex era in which we live, especially in this industry that changes as we breathe. Giving people some perspective helps. In fact, in the business world outside of health care, most clients are no longer in the same corporate structure they were in when we met them. They have either merged, acquired, been acquired, downsized, reengineered, or in general changed their shape, size, and structure. Health care is certainly not immune. Some hospitals we have worked with have been under a succession of three or four different corporate banners. Just when they learn one set of rules, expectations, and norms, they are sold and have to learn new ones. Anxiety is an ever-present companion. The constancy of this change is enough to intimidate any staff. Job security is history. You are asking people to commit more of themselves, with resources that may not be commensurate, to a future that is replete with question marks. Tall order! But that is where excellent leadership comes in, and where we see it practiced.

There are specific behaviors a leader can engage in to help others adapt. For starters, it helps to model personal and professional growth and nimbleness. Explain policies, procedures, or structural changes. Keep the information vacuum to a minimum. Help all employees understand that organizational, personal, financial, and emotional survival depend on growing, changing, letting go of the old, and embracing the new.

The imperative of adaptation is a message that must be delivered—in word and deed—from the highest rafters. Survival requires adaptation. Preach it, teach it, screech it. Individual employees and your organization as a whole will survive and thrive only by capitalizing on change and using it as an ally or competitive edge. Some employees will be unable to get beyond their own fears and doubts to make the necessary adaptations. Help these frightened people realize that change is their lifeboat.

Create an Environment That Questions Assumptions, Systems, and Processes

Tied to the whole issue of the emotional side of change is the reality of making adjustments, discarding the obsolete, and implementing new structures. You do not advocate change for change's sake, but you do want to create an environment that does not protect sacred cows. Woven into the fabric of your organization should be an environment that rewards those who question the status quo. Setting up that mentality as a norm can help carve out excellence in all you do. It suggests that each procedure, practice, or position must have a reason for being and make a positive contribution. Whatever does not meet those criteria finds itself in the rethink, redeploy, or remodel category.

One administrator of patient care services sees this process of questioning assumptions and challenging stereotypes as central to her role. She continually helps her mostly male colleagues on the executive staff realize that nurses have a bigger part on the caregiver team than that of the stereotypical nursing role—steady nurturer. She also challenges their assumption that her only job is that of advocate for nurses by demonstrating her concern for the entire organization and by showing a strong financial acumen that focuses on the bottom line.

Excellent leadership also teaches people who challenge the status quo that they have a responsibility to do their homework. They need not only to find the flaws but also to suggest fixes. Offering something better separates the serious problem solver from the disgruntled naysayer. Creating that mind-set is your best chance to tap the talent and commitment of all employees. Like a self-cleaning oven, it will keep you in good condition at all times.

Encourage Risks and Breaking New Ground

In times of great change, people often duck or head for cover. Rather than being visible by taking risks, employees try to stay unobtrusive and fade into the woodwork. That is not a behavior that leaders want to encourage. Safety may feel good, even though it is a mirage, but risk-averse behavior does not help the organization grow and remain competitive.

Kaiser Foundation Health Plan in Southern California encouraged risks, broke new ground, and paid attention to diversity and change all at the same time. Realizing the competitive nature of the health care climate, and understanding the need to groom people and help them reach their potential, Elizabeth Wu, the person in charge of the mentoring program, wanted to design something that would use resources efficiently while also achieving the goals of developing people for increased responsibility and growth. With these considerations in mind, she created a novel program, one half of which functions like the traditional mentoring program, with mentors matched to protégés, one-on-one. The part of Wu's program that broke new ground utilized a protégé group, all of whom were trying to learn or grow in both similar and different ways as they helped and learned from one another. One mentor facilitated the group, but the agenda and the areas for focus were determined by the protégés themselves. (More detailed information on this program is provided in Chapter Nine, because we get so many questions about mentoring.)

The point of the program is not that it was successful or unsuccessful, but rather that Elizabeth felt she could break a mold, take a risk, try something new, and make a flexible enough structure to meet individual and organizational goals at the same time despite all the constraints forced upon her.

Invest in Relationships with People Throughout the Industry, Organization, and Community

The need to deal well with people is not new, but doing so is just not universally practiced. Health care tends to see patients and families in high-stress situations that ultimately can add pressure to the staff. But in health care and every other field there is no substitute for good relationships. John D. Rockefeller once said that he would pay more for the ability to deal with people than for any commodity under the sun.[8] Smart man. You can surround yourself with talent, knowledge, intellect, and vision; but to capture the hearts and minds of the employees and the patients you serve at important times in their lives, you must demonstrate your own strengths while simultaneously acknowledging, valuing, respecting, and using theirs.

Effective health care leaders continue to tell us how many hours they spend serving on governmental task forces, boards of directors of community agencies, and industry association committees. These quasi-social activities build important relationships into the various geographical and professional ethnic communities important to the institution. One CEO of an inner-city hospital serving a large population of indigent and poor used connections in the community to raise enough funds to build a brand-new, state-of-the-art emergency room for an almost totally immigrant population that can often seem ignored by formal health care channels in an era of tight resources. Building good relationships with those who have both formal and informal influence within a given health care community is good business.

Leadership Fulfilled: Steps Toward Lasting Change

Having worked with hundreds of clients in and out of health care over the last twenty years, we have seen more fits and starts that ultimately stalled than we have seen successful completions of cultural change. To be sure, in most cases the leaders who envisioned the change had, like the proverbial road to hell, very good intentions, but for legitimate, and sometimes not so legitimate, reasons substantial, enduring, and successful completion of change eluded the organization. That does not mean that nothing good occurred through the change process, nor does it mean that because objectives usually changed from those originally stated, the change itself was not satisfactorily concluded. However, when we look at organizations that started out with clarity, determination, commitment, and focus to reach their marathon goal of creating an inclusive culture throughout the organization, most have fallen short. The reasons for disappointing conclusions vary from changing priorities midstream to failing to understand the complexity of the issues to not fully grasping the consequences of any significant change. Whatever the reasons, the results left people wanting, and frequently created a bigger trust vacuum.

For example, we remember one young, dynamic health care organization that was growing rapidly. It had among its prime visions an environment for its employees that was welcoming and inclusive, and it had as a goal matching the staff to the population it served. For that reason, the organization called us to do a full-blown diversity program. The initial impetus was the exclusion felt by members of the employee gay and lesbian coalition. The CEO wanted no one to feel left out. He was sensitive and smart enough to understand that any lack of commitment by an employee for whatever reason watered down productivity and performance.

After several meetings with some impressive, committed, and dynamic members of the staff, we began planning, educating, strategizing, and building a leadership team that would assume responsibility for the cultural change effort.

Simultaneously to the diversity effort, this young and confident organization was branching out across the United States and acquiring new facilities. We started to notice that meeting time was harder and harder to come by, and that executive-level presence and visibility were waning. When meetings repeatedly got postponed and we were unable to deliver services for which we had been paid, we kept leaving messages with our vice-presidential-level contact. When we finally caught up with him by phone, he said he did not want us thinking that diversity was not a priority because it was, but "of the organization's top twenty-five priorities, diversity is number twenty-four." That was our last conversation.

In contrast, one CEO, Mark Meyers, who we previously mentioned, is successful at overseeing and accomplishing long-term change. We first met Meyers when he was CEO for what was then AMI's Garden Grove Hospital. It was approximately eight years ago that we worked with him and his staff to implement a guest relations program, and long after Mark and many of the other key players left, that program is still going strong. The excellence in the structure and design of the program itself was not so rare. We have seen other good designs, effective training, and some integration into existing systems through quality improvement teams. But what makes Garden Grove's program unique is its longevity and its conversion of excellent service into the culture and bone marrow of the organization. For this reason, we interviewed Mark to see if he could identify elements of that particular guest relations program that could be applied to other long-term cultural change efforts, particularly around diversity.[9]

For starters, it is important to understand Mark's organization when he was in Santa Ana and to put it in context for the purpose of understanding the soil in which its beginning diversity efforts are being planted. The Santa Ana community has been predominantly

Hispanic since the mid-1970s. As a result, public policy has been to provide prenatal, obstetric, and pediatric care for undocumented immigrants because their children will be United States citizens. Because it has served such a large Hispanic population, Santa Ana has always hired a substantial number of Hispanic employees. As the demographics of the area have changed, there has been an increased need to reach out to the Vietnamese and Cambodian populations for hiring as well, but to date it has been very difficult to find Vietnamese nurses.

As an incentive for all staff to be more sensitive to diversity issues, employees can get a $500 bonus for passing a test of minimal Spanish competency. There is, however, no hourly differential for being bilingual. Language competency, like so many other potentially volatile diversity conundrums, can become a hot-button issue for staff. For example, Mark shared a story of a switchboard operator who could not speak Spanish. A non-English-speaking person from the community called the switchboard and said in Spanish, "I'm bleeding." The operator did not understand so she could not be helpful or understand the urgency of the situation. Although the hospital avoided a calamity in that particular event, Meyers realized from that experience that in a hospital whose patient base is 60 percent Hispanic, two-thirds of whom speak only that language, switchboard operators must be bilingual. Two long-term, tenured employees were given the option of learning Spanish but they did not want to. It was a tough call but he had to let them go. He justified his decision by saying that when demographics change, so does the job description. Taking a clear stand on visible issues and making tough calls is part of what leadership is all about.

Meyers knows full well that some monolingual staff resented not only that decision but also the fact that bilingual people get hiring preference when two candidates are equally qualified. In an attempt to level the playing field a little and help everyone, Meyers has offered Spanish classes with a gifted language instructor named Bill Harvey. His "Spanish for Gringos" class can assist in giving non-Spanish-speaking employees willing to learn a new language the ability to at least greet and be minimally conversant with their patients. Understanding the language just a little increases knowledge of the culture a lot and makes employees more aware and sensitive. That is the good news. The reality, however, is that some employees have a hard time getting beyond the resentment of having to learn another language at all.

Meyers's leadership can be seen in other ways that try to increase intercultural sensitivity. Visiting hours are more accommodating for people with special needs, and waiting rooms are designed to be bigger and more flexible, to make room for extended families. Meyers encourages physicians and hospital personnel to pay attention to culturally appropriate greetings as a way to welcome people to what could be an intimidating institution. For example, he suggests that when meeting members of a Hispanic family the hospital staff should do a subtle bow, shake hands starting with the oldest male, and say "mucho gusto" to everyone. To recall an old song, "Little things mean a lot."

In bolstering his business case argument for paying attention to diversity, Meyers tells about the success of some physicians as a result of attention paid to diversity. He notes that doctors of Asian and Middle Eastern backgrounds have very busy practices. The Hispanic community has welcomed them and helped them to build their practices because they treat patients with respect and without condescension. The busiest obstetrician serving the community is a doctor from Thailand. Meyers attributes this flourishing practice to the sensitivity of the doctor and his unwillingness to forget what it is like to feel like an outsider. Meyers also talks about a physician who came from Italy years ago who has never forgotten what it felt like to adapt and acculturate. This doctor's empathy and sensitivity have been central to his building a very successful practice.

Of course life is not nirvana at Santa Ana anymore than it is elsewhere. There are the predictable cultural differences and examples of physician abruptness that cause conflict. In those instances, effective leadership necessitates direct feedback with clear consequences. When, for example, a foreign-born-and-trained physician made comments regarding a female employee that on the basis of his cultural perception he viewed as harmless dialogue but that she defined as harassment on the basis of hers, Meyers's feedback was direct with clear consequences: "If you do or say that again, this will be the result."

Through the primary care council at Santa Ana, young physician recruits are coached, counseled, and trained to understand the community they are serving. This crash course can be preemptive and help the recruits avoid any problems that would result in a CEO issuing an ultimatum. The primary care council helps the young doctors with some specific suggestions that are obvious to the culturally literate but that may be less obvious to the uninitiated. The concreteness of these suggestions can be helpful. Some examples are

- You need bilingual staff, and as much as possible you as a doctor should enhance bilingual capabilities.

- Cater to the whole family, not just to the patient.

- Have waiting rooms that are three to five times bigger than you originally thought of to accommodate the families.

- Be careful not to speak your own language with a coworker in front of people who do not understand it.

Some physicians get frustrated when these suggestions are made, and on occasion Meyers is shocked at their narrow-mindedness. But he has determined that his leadership can be useful in helping doctors be successful, and he is trying to get them up to speed so they will avoid the land mines before them.

Meyers also believes that cultural sensitivity is a two-way street and he tries to make that clear. Certainly there is a need to increase everyone's sensitivity, starting with Anglos who are serving pluralistic populations. But the need does not end there. Meyers has observed that frequently those who have been in this country ten or more years tend to forget what it felt like when they first came. They lose not only their sensitivity but also their patience for the unacculturated. Finally, the responsibility for learning also falls on the newcomers. They need to understand why their behaviors may be creating resentment, and they need to understand the practices and norms of their new community. Using cultural interpreters, people who are truly bicultural, to explain the whys and wherefores is helpful.

Adaptation and acculturation are two-way streets. Any CEO or executive staff of a medical operation today who wants to make diversity an asset will at sometime wrestle with this balance. In the next chapter we focus on ways to educate the community. For now, it is important to contemplate how a leader shapes the internal organization and holds people across the board accountable for managing their cross-cultural issues successfully.

Meyers has identified six critical steps in any long-term change effort. As we discuss each, think about diversity efforts in your organization and ask the hard questions.

1. *Design and customize a program, do not impose it.* The most effective long-term change efforts are tailored to the uniquenesses and realities of a given organization. In HMOs, for example, with multiple sites and locations, effective change occurs when it is customized to suit the particular needs of each location. Receptivity to change depends on many things, not the least of which is perception of control rather than perception of imposition. Customizing can be a great asset in opening people's minds and minimizing their resistance.

2. *Tailor reward systems.* Leaders should make it a goal to teach people, with as much specificity and concreteness as possible, to be successful in these systems, and to consistently reinforce the behaviors the leader wants. This goal is most successfully and consistently accomplished by using performance reviews to articulate expectations clearly and hold employees accountable. The rewards that follow can range from pats on the back to promotions, chances for new opportunities or letters of commendation. Matching the reward as closely as possible to something the rewarded values is

helpful. You do not want to publicly commend someone who would be embarrassed by it, but a quiet thank you or a note of appreciation could mean a great deal.

3. *Managers embrace the issue and model the behavior.* At Garden Grove, the managers modeled the importance of the program in ways big and small, serious and fun. Instead of being cynical about one more initiative, the managers led, supported, role-modeled, and reinforced the importance of good guest relations. For example, the motto of the guest relations program was "Our care shows." Managers could send out CareGrams (telegram-like written compliments) to employees caught doing the right things. Care dollars also could be awarded and employees could get $5 bonuses. For Halloween, staff dressed in costume and the usual "Our Care Shows" buttons were replaced by ones that said "Our Scare Grows."

4. *The change must be measurable.* Garden Grove has moved from the bottom third to the top third of AMI hospitals on the basis of patient feedback. Every year the hospital sent a questionnaire to patients that focused on improving one aspect of its performance. Through intense, clear focus, through management support, and through utilization of rewards and reinforcement, one indicator at a time, they improved each year.

5. *The initiative is bigger than any individual.* This point is critical. We have seen numerous organizations in which an initiative has a tremendous launch and a long trajectory. Then its primary champion leaves, and like a balloon that has been punctured the initiative deflates and erodes. The only way to avoid this danger is to build the changes into the systems themselves and get ownership at every level of the organization at every step along the way. One hospital achieved this with its guest relations program. The managers designed the mission statement and motto, identified the behaviors they wanted reinforced, and conceived the desired goals. They even tailored the language they wanted to the measuring tools used. The structure of the process and feedback seeped into every level of the organization. The end result was that when two

of the top executives left, the program remained intact and fully able to continue.

6. *Build rewards and consequences into new-employee orientation.* It is easier to create and reinforce the culture you want by shaping employee behavior at the beginning than to try to change habits later. Provide expectations and rules up front. Explain how these behaviors will be part of performance reviews. The more specific you are, the better. For example, a clear expectation might be, "Don't speak a language in front of a patient that he or she doesn't understand." Then, when employees are sensitive to language issues, use positive reinforcement. Thank yous and acknowledgment of good work help. Ultimately, demonstrating consequences when undesirable behavior occurs is also necessary.

7. *There is no substitute for ethical behavior.* The exploration of what constitutes ethical behavior is becoming more and more of a focus in organizations of all industries. Our colleague Patricia Digh recently wrote an article in *HRM Magazine* in which she illustrated the complexity of ethics, particularly as it relates to cross-cultural issues. Digh quotes a number of noted writers and thinkers in the field. One of them, Michael Daigneault, president of the Washington, D.C.–based Ethics Resource Center, calls ethics "the glue that holds the company together and defines it as an entity." Companies are known and defined not only by the products and services they deliver, he said, but also by the way they provide those products and services.[10]

Rushworth Kidder, president of the Camden, Maine–based Institute for Global Ethics, suggests that real ethical dilemmas and choices show themselves not in right versus wrong situations but, rather, in right versus right.[11] For a health care example, consider where organizations choose to spend their limited resources. On one hand you have Dr. Jack Kevorkian espousing physician-assisted suicide. Although that view gives most of us great pause, particularly physicians, who have taken the Hippocratic oath, the reality, on the other hand, is not always so clear. Just look at a few other ethical dilemmas in health care:

- What are the criteria to be a recipient on an organ donor list?
  How are the tough decisions made about who gets the heart?
  The answer literally influences who might live and who might
  die among a whole list of deserving patients.
- How much of an institution's limited resources should be
  devoted to neonatal care for babies who weigh a pound, or at
  the other end of life, on elderly who have no chance of a
  meaningful future life?
- Does legal or illegal immigrant status have any impact on
  who gets services? If you see someone in dire need of care, is
  he simply a human being in need, or some foreigner who is a
  drain on a community?

That ethical clashes do and will continue to exist is as predictable as night and day. But here is where an organization's values
can act as a moral compass. The research of Rushworth Kidder,
mentioned earlier, from the Institute for Global Ethics, reveals five
core human values across cultures: compassion, fairness, honesty,
responsibility, and respect for others.[12] The challenge for leaders,
and the opportunity, is to operationalize these values across cultural
lines. What is interesting about Kidder's research is that participants
represented 143 countries and more than fifty faiths. These top five
values were arrived at by giving respondents a list of seventeen values and asking them to rate core values and what would matter
most in the future.

Kidder's perception is that these values go not to the core of
what it means to be American, Salvadoran, or Chilean, but rather
to the core of what it means to be human. For the leader in any
health care organization, but particularly one that is serving a pluralistic organization, ethical behavior is at the top of what it means
to be a respected leader.

For example, many Catholic health care organizations count
among their core values respect. This value translates into a policy
of nondiscrimination, even, for example, to employees or patients
who may be gay or lesbian. Each organization and its leaders need

to rely on the organization's core values to steer the course of moral choices. To see where ethical dilemmas have an impact on your organization, spend some time on the assessment provided in Exhibit 7.1. Have any of the pressures listed in this assessment ever caused employees to break the rules? When they do, what are the consequences? If a rule is broken once, what happens the next time the same dilemma is faced?

If we take the optimist's point of view, the one that presumes that most people want to behave ethically but they just need a little help, we can again refer to what Patricia Digh calls the warning signs.[13] You know you are in trouble ethically if one of the following thoughts is a frequent mental or verbal companion of yours. If it is, just give it a ✓:

❑ 1. "Well, maybe just this once."

❑ 2. "No one will ever know."

❑ 3. "Everyone does it."

❑ 4. "It doesn't matter how it gets done as long as it gets done."

❑ 5. Other _____

❑ 6. Other _____

Most human beings can probably check off all of these at one time or another, and the third item seems to be a perpetual part of pubescence. The question is, how can leaders help people grow beyond these rather human but unethical rationalizations?

None of us has fully arrived at the highest ethical standards, but in leading teams, organizations, communities, or countries, high ethical standards do matter. They are even more complex and critical when people come together in pluralistic health care organizations, where definitions of right and wrong will undoubtedly vary due to differing cultural norms. Again, we refer to a set of questions that Digh suggests we ask and use as a guide to helping all employees enhance their ethical behavior:[14]

EXHIBIT 7.1 Ethics and You.

Directions: Think about your organization's standards as well as about your own standards for ethical behavior. Once you have done that, put a check mark next to any of the following pressures that cause you to violate those standards.

Pressures	The Organization's Standards	Your Own Standards
Fulfilling schedules and deadlines	❏	❏
Meeting aggressive financial or business objectives	❏	❏
Helping the company survive	❏	❏
Advancing the career interests of my boss	❏	❏
Peer pressure	❏	❏
Resisting competitive threats	❏	❏
Saving jobs (mine or others)	❏	❏
Advancing my own career or financial interests	❏	❏
Representing the hospital/medical center to the target community	❏	❏

Source of Pressures: Ethics Resource Center, *Ethics in American Business: Politics, Programs and Perceptions* (Washington, D.C.: Ethics Resource Center, 1994), p. 21. Reprinted by permission.

1. Are my actions legal?
2. Will my actions stand the test of time?
3. How would it look in the newspaper (or in the light of day anywhere)?
4. Will I sleep soundly tonight?
5. What would I tell my child to do? Would what I tell my child be consistent with my actions?

We know that conversations about ethics are shaded in multiple hues of gray. We are not saying that making ethical decisions is easy, nor are we saying that behaviors and choices are exact. What we are saying is that anyone who leads a health care organization of any sort in this day and age has to be willing to start the dialogue and engage in the exploration of multiple, complex issues. When we talk to employees about leadership, the biggest turn off and trust buster is hypocrisy, double standards, not "walking the talk," not being authentic. Ethics is not an elite, remote topic; it is a practical, daily issue. It is about who individuals are; it is about what an organization's values, norms, mores, and morals are; and it is about how organizations behave or make choices that are consistent with their beliefs and values. Leadership that ultimately builds trust and fosters credibility will necessitate leadership that has a strong sense of organizational values and a code of conduct, policies, and behaviors that are consistent with these values. This chapter has looked at leadership in a number of ways, and it has suggested ingredients necessary to accomplish long-term change, with the goal of achieving diversity objectives.

The one thought you can take to the bank regarding leadership is that guiding an organization through a long-term process is complex. It requires understanding, vision, energy, tenacity, adaptability, integrity, sensitivity, and passion, to name just a few necessary qualities. Add to any ordinarily complex change the specific task of culture change around diversity and that change might appear daunting. But it is doable. It can be infinitely rewarding financially and emotionally. In a nod to Darwin's survival-of-the-fittest theory, we suggest that the organizations and leaders who survive today's battles will be those with the courage and determination to embark on this potentially rewarding but undeniably challenging opportunity.

8

Overcoming Barriers to Change

If you have read the chapters in this book sequentially, you have received, we hope, some new information and have begun to wrestle with complex problems that illustrate a dynamic health care industry at the end of the second millennium. Although you may have little control over the pace and the magnitude of change, you do have options about how you and your organization can manage that change and make it work. To capitalize on diversity as part of an overall strategy, three areas of change need to be attended to simultaneously: individual attitudes and beliefs, managerial-staff relations, and organizational systems (see Figure 8.1).

The first area, *individual attitudes and beliefs*, affects interpersonal interactions at every level of the organization. Examining this area involves looking at how employees feel about the changes in the health care industry, and how staff feel about serving or accommodating patients and their families who have very different norms. It also involves looking at the assumptions individuals have about various professional groups on staff or about cultural groups in the community.

Managerial-staff relations are among the most significant determiners of how employees feel about their organization. Productivity, tenacity, and commitment are often influenced by one's relationship to a manager or direct supervisor. For this reason, helping your upwardly mobile staff develop appropriate skills is critical. Team building, problem solving, conflict resolution, and coaching

are examples of skills that are essential to being an effective manager in any setting, but even more so during the rapid change that
is taking place throughout the health care industry.

Finally, the positive results that progressive organizations seek
turn on *organizational systems*. Neither the most far-reaching, enlightened individual nor the most highly developed managerial skills
and practices will produce meaningful change in an organization if
its systems and policies do not foster, reward, and hold people
accountable for the values, norms, and behaviors an organization is
promoting as its way of being in and doing business. A hospital or
clinic that wants to capitalize on diversity must probe its business
assumptions. For starters, think about how diversity is perceived as
a strategic asset. Also consider how organizational policies either
encourage or discourage the attainment of an open, welcoming culture. To do so, get feedback about how diversity-friendly the values,
norms, and policies are to both internal and external customers.

Making Your Diversity Efforts Pay Off

When these three areas—beliefs, interpersonal relations, and systems—work in concert, diversity can become a strategic asset. The
question is, how do you make it so? If it were easy, most organizations would already be doing it. The steps outlined in this chapter
will not only give you some clues as to what is needed but will also
expose some gaps. In these gaps are the signs of both sabotage and
success. The seven steps we are about to discuss are designed to help
any committed organization understand the stages of a process that
is truly continuous and evolutionary. The continuous part is not
designed to be overwhelming, but rather to create realistic expectations that the process is long, contains unplanned detours, and
includes goals, plans, and commitment that may change midstream.
With that sober reality as a backdrop, diversity leaders and imple-
menters know that good things can and do come from a well-
thought-out, well-designed strategic change process. This chapter
explains how.

Figure 8.1 Capitalizing on Diversity: Three Arenas of Focus.

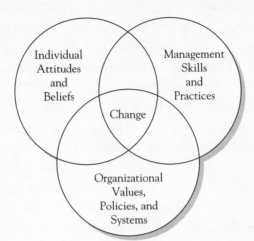

Get Commitment from the Top

The perception that commitment from the top is critical is common knowledge. Almost everyone who works in an organization knows that to embark on any long-term change, particularly one that has the baggage that diversity carries, necessitates visible, symbolic, and real commitment from the top. If staff perceive that executives are just going through the motions, employees will too, and they will resent the work they cannot finish because they have to attend meetings or training sessions on behalf of some empty gesture. Executives must actually *be* earnest, not just feel pressured by the latest "flavor of the month." Beyond feeling a strong commitment, top leadership needs to "walk the talk." We already mentioned the necessity for this in our discussion of ethics and integrity in the previous chapter, but it bears repeating. *An organization is better off never starting the work of diversity than starting it and dropping it at the first new crisis, change in priority, or budget crunch.*

A hopeful example is the city of San Diego, which early in the 1990s, at the height of California's recession, committed itself to a culture that eliminated racism and sexism and encouraged equity and an appreciation of all employees. Municipalities throughout the state were strapped, but even in the face of economic hurdles San Diego city government hung tough and provided four days of training for all managers and supervisors. The organizational development (OD) branch, who did this work at the instigation of the city manager, were somewhat skeptical. The OD staff would not take any bets on how long the initiative would last when money got tighter, but they and the rest of the government staff were pleasantly surprised when the city manager chose to honor its commitment. That is what employees need to see from top executives.

They also need to see executives talk about diversity face to face, and to listen to their leaders describe why it is a strategic imperative. Above all, employees need to see, and have demonstrated, that the executives are accountable along with the rest of the organization. Diversity leaders do not do what one client did, which was to have the CEO preach about hiring and promoting more diverse candidates, yet every time an opening appeared and a group of very competent candidates applied from a wide variety of backgrounds, only white males seemed to make the cut.

Staff will be understandably skeptical of diversity initiatives until they see this commitment tested. Are diversity efforts abandoned when there is a budget crunch? Are executives too busy to attend sessions and hear staff's perceptions about obstacles? The answers to these and similar questions will send a clear message, and behavior will always be believed over words. As Ralph Waldo Emerson wrote, "I can't hear what you're saying because what you are rings so loudly in my ears." Actions not only speak loudly, they scream.

As you consider ways to get commitment from the top, mull over the following questions to see if anything can dampen your efforts to recruit top-level support:

- What is going on in your organization that could vie for the resources, attention, and support needed for a diversity initiative?

- How have executives previously demonstrated commitment on other important issues? What is their track record of making good on promises?

- How much do top-level staff really understand diversity? Are they aware of any of their own biases and assumptions? Are they interested in exploring them?

- What is the level of trust and good will in your organization? How do you know? State some of the indicators. What has leadership done—be specific here—to create the climate you currently see?

Answer these questions, or at least ponder them, as a first step in getting insight into what you might be able to expect from leadership.

Then answer the ten questions in Exhibit 8.1 and look at the results. The more "I can count on it" answers you have, the easier it will be to solidify commitment. If you have a lot of "Not sure" answers, you have some homework to do. If most of your responses clearly fall under the umbrella of "You've got to be kidding," then getting executive commitment could be a long, hard haul.

We end this section with one more example. Several years ago we facilitated a national diversity forum for the Society of Human Resource Management. One of our speakers was from Federal Express. That company at that time had an outstanding diversity initiative that was all the more unique in that it was a grassroots effort. Diversity looks different at every level of an organization, and one of the things that employees at Federal Express did is get their CEO's attention. If need be, each organization will have to decide how to do that in its own way. We said you need commitment from the top; we did not say you have to start there to get it.

Assess and Diagnose

"Know thyself" is as important a dictum for organizations as it is for individuals. Before a company can figure out how to make diversity

EXHIBIT 8.1 Testing Commitment from the Top.

Directions: Read the items below and put check marks in the appropriate columns.

Item	I can count on it	Not sure	You've got to be kidding
Our CEO and other executives talk frequently about diversity's strategic importance.	❑	❑	❑
Our leadership team models appreciation of diversity in its membership.	❑	❑	❑
Visible support is shown in speeches, newsletters, and other communication vehicles.	❑	❑	❑
Leadership tries to understand diversity issues in our organization by taking time to talk to employees at all levels.	❑	❑	❑
Sensitivity is demonstrated through flextime policies.	❑	❑	❑
Holidays, symbols, celebrations, and rituals of many groups are honored and respected here.	❑	❑	❑
There are many ways to do things here, not just one.	❑	❑	❑
The performance review of all employees acknowledges diversity.	❑	❑	❑
Top leadership demonstrates knowledge of different cultural norms in its behavior.	❑	❑	❑
Executive members serve on task force teams and/or attend training to demonstrate commitment.	❑	❑	❑

a competitive advantage, it needs to assess existing conditions; analyze barriers to productivity, inclusion, and commitment; and clearly articulate a set of goals and measures that identify criteria for success.

Assessment and diagnosis start with a good look inward that helps staff at all levels clarify who the organization is (its values), what it is about (its mission), and where it wants to go (its vision). Beyond these discussions lies the opportunity to influence the organizational processes and systems to help achieve the desired goals and potential.

To know what systems need tinkering and what skills and awarenesses need to be taught requires data. Meaningful culture change is data driven. Data are the information that influences and confirms the diagnosis and legitimizes any effort on which you embark.

A combination of interviews, focus groups, and questionnaires can be used to gather data for analysis. The analysis of data is then shared with senior management. It should provide a description of existing conditions as well as strategies to deal with diversity issues.

The chart in Table 8.1 elaborates the advantages and disadvantages of a number of ways of collecting data. What makes one method appropriate over another depends on many things, such as cost, time, organizational history, number of languages in which data are collected, and the various cultures represented on staff, to name a few. The appropriateness of which style of data collection to use in soliciting feedback is often culturally influenced.

It is worth noting that not all data have to be collected in formal ways. Through meetings and other formats, questionnaires that are quick and easy to complete can be distributed. For example, suppose the human resources department would like to find out how employees see customer service. The sample tool provided in Exhibit 8.2 might work fine. The higher the overall point total is, the more effectively the hospital is serving its patients. What may be even more telling, however, than the overall total is the score for

TABLE 8.1 Feedback Method Compared.

Method	Advantages	Disadvantages
Questionnaire	Data can be obtained from customers in a cost-effective way.	Requires literacy and possibly translations into other languages. Takes time that people may not want to give. Also, not a norm in some cultures and may be too intimidating.
	Data are collected quickly in ways that can be analyzed easily.	One-way communication offers no way to get clarification or explanation about responses.
	Data from all respondents are provided in comparative form so they can be quantified and statistically analyzed.	Responses tend to be limited by information requested in questionnaire.
	Can be done simultaneously in many locations.	May get lip service and perfunctory answers that respondents think the bank wants to hear rather than thoughtful responses.
	Is simple to administer.	Impersonality and lack of human touch may put off customers from relationship-oriented cultures.
Interviews	Interviewees may feel freer to speak openly without others present.	Least time-efficient and most costly method.
	Problems and issues surfaced can be explored in depth.	Requires skilled interviewer to guide sessions.
	Permits collection of examples, anecdotes, and stories that illustrate the issues and put them in human terms.	Data collected from a limited number of people may provide a narrow slice of information if only staff at certain levels are interviewed.

| | | For bilingual interviews, you need a skilled bilingual, bicultural interviewer to get good data. |

More personal touch allows for one-on-one communication.

Focus Groups — Serve as a teaching tool, building respondents' awareness about the process in question.

In-depth discussions about topics and issues yield richer data.

Two-way communication permits clarification and explanation of information.

Is more personal and human.

Subtle information can be picked up from nonverbal clues and body language.

Is more time-efficient to get information from groups rather than from individuals one at a time.

Interaction generates more data. Comments spark other ideas so new information may emerge.

Participants' hearing of each other's views may expand their understanding of the issues.

For bilingual interviews, you need a skilled bilingual, bicultural interviewer to get good data.

Require skilled facilitation in sessions and possibly bilingual facilitators.

Generally only get a sample of views, not everyone's.

Peer pressure may influence participants' comments.

Takes time to coordinate sessions and schedule the pulling of employees from jobs.

People may be uncomfortable in a new setting and an unfamiliar experience.

Participants may be reticent to open up and speak freely. Cultural norms may discourage negative or critical comments.

Need to have something in it for the consumers who are giving up their time.

Source: Lee Gardenswartz and Anita Rowe, *Managing Diversity: A Complete Desk Reference and Planning Guide* (Burr Ridge, Ill.: Irwin, 1993), p. 266. Reprinted by permission of *The Western Journal of Medicine.*

each of the three aspects. These scores will show, for example, whether services offered match the needs of the community, what systems in the medical center support and reinforce culturally competent care, and the nature of relationships among employees, and between employees and patients. Such data will indicate in which of these areas the organization excels and in which it needs to improve. The lowest scored items suggest where leaders should begin working to increase effectiveness.

A feedback tool that looks at the entire change process is the Managing Diversity Questionnaire presented in Exhibit 8.3. This tool mirrors the three areas mentioned at the beginning of the chapter and can be helpful as a full organizational scan. Data from this questionnaire could provide a task force with a blueprint of where the obstacles and issues are. Then the challenge would be to prioritize which outcomes it wants to start achieving.

After you have thought about these sample questionnaires and about the advantages and disadvantages of various methods listed in Table 8.1, consider a few more questions:

Are there existing data on hand that are current and valid? If so, use whatever data you have. If you need to augment the most recent culture audit with focus groups to more fully understand the nuances and complexity of the issues, set them up.

If you follow up an audit with focus groups for example, how are you cutting the groups? By that we mean, Are there some all-male and all-female groups? Do some groups include only English speakers and some those who speak only Tagalog? Have you kept participants in job-alike groups or at the same levels? We have seen single-parent groups, union groups, gay and lesbian groups, and groups of older workers. There is no right or wrong way to slice the groups, but you should have some strategic reason for whatever cuts you make.

Pay attention to the rumor mill. What is the overall response to the process of data collection? Are staff cynical? Perhaps some are excited to speak up, while others are convinced that this effort will amount to nothing, like so many before it have. You need to address

EXHIBIT 8.2 Serving Diverse Patients and Families: An Assessment Questionnaire.

Directions: Rate your hospital by placing a check mark in the appropriate column.

	Very True	Sometimes True	Not True
1. We learn about the customs of others to meet the needs of our patients.	☐	☐	☐
2. We have alternate methods of communicating with and helping our patients.	☐	☐	☐
3. Resources are spent to educate employees about the cross-cultural norms of our community population.	☐	☐	☐
4. We solicit and get feedback from patients about their treatment and care.	☐	☐	☐
5. Employees are rewarded for specific behaviors that make people feel welcome.	☐	☐	☐
6. Patients are treated with dignity and respect.	☐	☐	☐
7. We are aware of the genetic predispositions of the populations we serve.	☐	☐	☐
8. Employees are encouraged to find ways to respect the traditions and beliefs of all the patients.	☐	☐	☐
9. Employees have good interpersonal communication skills.	☐	☐	☐
10. We know enough about the needs and preferences of community members to offer patient care in appropriate fashion.	☐	☐	☐
11. We have people to consult as resources when we need to learn more.	☐	☐	☐
12. Hospital administrators participate in community organizations and functions.	☐	☐	☐
13. Management spends time learning new skills to manage a wider array of people.	☐	☐	☐
14. We have alternative ways to help people in crisis.	☐	☐	☐

EXHIBIT 8.2 Serving Diverse Patients and Families: An Assessment Questionnaire, *continued.*

	Very True	Sometimes True	Not True
15. Employees have been trained in customer service and communication skills.	☐	☐	☐
16. We can effectively accommodate non-English speakers.	☐	☐	☐
17. Management has made it clear that diversity is a top priority.	☐	☐	☐
18. Employees are open to serving ethnic populations different from their own.	☐	☐	☐

Scoring: Very true = 2 points
          Sometimes true = 1 point
          Not true = 0 points

Items 1, 4, 7, 10, 13, 16   Services   _____ Points

Items 2, 5, 8, 11, 14, 17   Systems   _____ Points

Items 3, 6, 9, 12, 15, 18   Relationships   _____ Points

                                Total Points   _____

EXHIBIT 8.3 Managing Diversity Questionnaire.

In this organization	Very True	Sometimes True	Not True
1. I am at ease with people of diverse backgrounds.	☐	☐	☐
2. There is diverse staff at all levels.	☐	☐	☐
3. Managers have a track record of hiring and promoting diverse employees.	☐	☐	☐
4. In general, I find change stimulating, exciting, and challenging.	☐	☐	☐
5. Racial, ethnic, and gender jokes are tolerated in the informal environment.	☐	☐	☐
6. Managers hold all people equally accountable.	☐	☐	☐
7. I know about the cultural norms of different groups.	☐	☐	☐
8. The formation of ethnic and gender support groups is encouraged.	☐	☐	☐
9. Managers are flexible, structuring benefits and rules that work for everyone.	☐	☐	☐
10. I am afraid to disagree with members of other groups for fear of being called prejudiced.	☐	☐	☐
11. There is a mentoring program that identifies and prepares women and people of color for promotion.	☐	☐	☐
12. Appreciation of differences can be seen in the rewards managers give.	☐	☐	☐
13. I feel that there is more than one right way to do things.	☐	☐	☐
14. Members of the nondominant group feel they belong.	☐	☐	☐
15. One criteria of a manager's performance review is developing the diversity of his or her staff.	☐	☐	☐
16. I think that diverse viewpoints make for creativity.	☐	☐	☐
17. There is high turnover among women and people of color.	☐	☐	☐
18. Managers give feedback and evaluate performance so employees don't lose face.	☐	☐	☐
19. I am aware of my own assumptions and stereotypes.	☐	☐	☐

EXHIBIT 8.3 Managing Diversity Questionnaire, *continued.*

	Very True	Sometimes True	Not True
20. Policies are flexible enough to accommodate everyone.	☐	☐	☐
21. Managers get active participation from all employees in meetings.	☐	☐	☐
22. I think there is enough common ground to hold staff together.	☐	☐	☐
23. The speaking of other languages is forbidden.	☐	☐	☐
24. Multicultural work teams function harmoniously.	☐	☐	☐
25. Staff members spend their lunch hour and breaks in mixed groups.	☐	☐	☐
26. Money and time are spent on diversity development activities.	☐	☐	☐
27. Managers effectively use problem-solving skills to deal with language differences or other culture clashes.	☐	☐	☐
28. I feel that working in a diverse staff enriches me.	☐	☐	☐
29. Top management backs up its value on diversity with action.	☐	☐	☐
30. Managers have effective strategies to use when one group refuses to work with another.	☐	☐	☐

Scoring:

Items 5, 10, 17, 23   Very true = 0 points   Somewhat = 1 point, Not true = 2 points

All other items   Very true = 2 points, Somewhat = 1 point, Not true = 0 points

_____ Individual attitudes and beliefs   Items 1,4,7,10,13,16,19,22,25,28

_____ Organizational values and norms   Items 2,5,8,11,14,17,20,23,26,29

_____ Management practices and policies   Items 3,6,9,12,15,18,21,24,27,30

_____ Total Score

Source: Lee Gardenswartz and Anita Rowe, *Managing Diversity: A Complete Desk Reference and Planning Guide* (Burr Ridge, Ill.: Irwin, 1993), pp. 268–269. Reprinted by permission of *The Western Journal of Medicine.*

these concerns so you can minimize the disruption and frustration at the intrusion of collecting data.

If you have recently collected information and done nothing with it, alarm bells should be going off in your head. Do not ask for feedback if you are not committed to using the data. And if your organization's past is checkered in the data-collection arena but you plan to do better this time around, be prepared for resistance and have a ready answer for the snide comments that will arise. Like the sun in the morning, they will come up.

Finally, consider the drawbacks to collecting these data. Among the issues to think about are the amount of time and money involved and the perceived relevance of the data. For the reluctant cynics in your organization, how can you minimize disruption, and what can you offer as a benefit of getting these data? Certainly busy employees and the organization need to think they will be better off for having participated. If these issues cannot be addressed satisfactorily, do not even think about starting.

Create the Diversity Task Force

Someone or some group needs to function as an advocate and shepherd of diversity initiatives. This person's or group's role should be to oversee the process and be accountable for its progress. A cross-functional, multilevel, diverse team committed to change, with representation from all parts of the organization, is generally the most credible and energetic. This task force first needs to be developed as a team and trained in diversity awareness, knowledge, and sensitivity. Once it has forged a collective sense of purpose, built cohesive interpersonal relationships, and spent time understanding each team member's assets and issues, the task force will be poised to formulate a plan for your hospital or medical center. This plan may include both training and systemic problem solving.

There are a number of excellent models for developing and utilizing a task force. The most common one we see is one that is efficient and practical, that gets people up to speed, builds good relationships for joint problem solving, and is effective.

Such a task force or council typically has two days of team training. Day one is designed to increase individual awareness about biases, culture, the organization's paradigm of diversity, the business case for diversity, and general content knowledge about the distinction between affirmative action, valuing differences, and managing diversity. In the process the council members increase their own awareness and group cohesion.

The next step is to formulate a diversity plan that will lead to the accomplishment of organizational goals. That plan often includes both training and systemic problem solving. Thus, day two of training sees the task force define its mission and choose the specific goals and objectives that arise from that mission. The beginning of serious planning and implementation take place on day two.

The two-day council launch is a plan that can work very well, but again there are a few questions to answer.

How are task force members selected? What criteria are you using? Are people hand picked, or are you looking for volunteers or a combination of the two? Each selection method has an upside and a downside, and none is inherently superior. The most critical issue is that task force members should collectively reflect your entire organization and have credibility.

What are the indicators of credibility in your organization? What would someone serving on the task force gain? Would peer pressure encourage or discourage serving?

What is the history of task forces where you work? Based on that history, what kind of prognosis is there for a good outcome?

Rather than close this section with questions, we want to make a few recommendations:

• Make sure the task force is clear about its parameters and its purpose. Is it a problem-solving body? Is it only a recommending body? What is the scope of its authority and its account-ability? There is no place for ambiguity around these questions.

- Keep in mind that for any problem that needs a solution there are many constituencies and vested interests.

- We cannot stress strongly enough how important it is that *all* constituencies be, and actually feel as though they are, represented in the task force.

- Make sure that data drive your initiative. In that data is the task force's legitimacy.

Problem Solve Systemic Issues

The problem solving of systemic issues is really the guts of any long-term change. Once the information about the climate has been gathered and diagnosed, it is important to solve substantive systemic problems and minimize obstacles. For example, questions may arise about the internal communication systems. Why is it taking so long to admit people and get them to their rooms? What departments are part of the admitting process? Is there a specific breakdown of the admitting process, or general laxness and inefficiency? Is there a breakdown in interdepartmental coordination? What needs to happen to ensure better communication and a smoother process between admitting, transportation, and housekeeping, for example?

Perhaps the communication dilemma is between medical center employees and patients. Are we serving a larger number of non-English-speaking patients? How many languages are we hearing? Do we have translators? If not, how can we communicate with our patients? If we do have translators, is that position a full-time job or are we pulling employees off of other work assignments to translate? What happens to their work that is not getting done? Should we pay them a differential for extra duty? If we do, will that cause resentment among other staff members? What on the surface seems like a systems issue around communication is very complicated and can affect hiring, profile, job descriptions, salary, and so on.

These are but a sample of the kinds of complex questions that need to be asked about whatever systems issues and questions are explored. Although there are numerous and different but effective ways to solve problems, whatever the process is, all methods involve asking and answering a few of the same questions.

Identify objectives and obstacles. What is our desired outcome? What are we trying to achieve? What are the gaps between the desired state and the current reality? Stated a little differently, what issues or obstacles exist that inhibit successful accomplishment of both long- and short-term goals?

Set criteria. If we achieve our desired goals, how will we know? What are the criteria, the markers, or the indicators of success? You cannot be too specific on this one. Concreteness and specificity are essential.

Brainstorm. Using the brainstorm process, come up with as many options as possible. Even the most outrageous ideas are worth considering.

Reality test. What possible steps are necessary to change the system? Who needs to be involved in the change? What does each party get out of maintaining the status quo? The answer to this question is critical because therein lies any motivation to resist change.

Follow-up and evaluate. Once you have determined a course of action, follow up; correct your course midstream as necessary and keep evaluating to see what is working and what is not. If you are meeting your criteria, there is a good chance your plan is working.

Any systems change is slow, painstaking work because the fixing of one problem is usually the birth of another. It helps to realize that glitches can be dealt with and changed, and that accountability can become a force that reshapes behavior. Often the biggest obstacles to being creative, effective problem solvers are the blocks that limit our ability to see options. Sir Edward DeBono, the creativity guru, suggested years ago that there are some problem-solving blocks that inhibit good outcomes. Some of these blocks cluster around the human need for order and pre-dictability. Among these blocks are the need to be right, the fear of failure (and of success), and the discomfort with ambiguity. Another kind of block has to do with belief systems, values, and attitudes. For example, what biases do you have regarding health care? What assumptions do you make about physicians, or wheel chairs, or the size and number of beds your local medical center has, or how high tech your medical center is? Finally, environ-mental blocks cause distraction, such as beepers or a room that is too big or too small, too hot or too cold.

Consider which blocks inhibit you from being your most cre-ative and open. Which do you see inhibiting your colleagues? Think about systems that most need fixing at your organization. Which of these blocks could get in the way of your collective suc-cess? What will each party get out of the change process? If you can-not figuratively stand in the shoes of an employee in facilities management or dietary or billing or lab and see what is in the solu-tion for each person, and if you cannot articulate that benefit to each department, getting employee buy-in will be difficult. Theo-retically, you want a solution that leaves everyone feeling positive.

Train to Address Awareness, Knowledge, and Skill Needs

Misunderstandings and differences can escalate and cause major conflicts if staff are not trained about cultural differences. Cultural knowledge and awareness, personal attitudes, beliefs and assump-tions, stereotypes, and management skill are all areas that can be developed and positively affected through training.

A most important question is, Why or under what conditions should you conduct diversity training? The following list may shed some light:

- When there are complaints about insensitive comments being made or jokes being told in the work unit about age, gender, ethnicity, sexual orientation, or physical ability.

- When you seem to be unable to retain members of diverse groups or, in fact, any employee you want to keep.

- When there is open conflict between people from different groups.

- When there is a lack of diversity throughout all levels of the organization.

- When cultural faux pas are committed out of ignorance, not out of malice.

- When there are complaints about language related to blocks in communication.

- When misinterpretation or failure to understand directions leads to mistakes, the repeating of tasks, and low productivity.

- When there are Equal Employment Opportunity Commission (EEOC) suits and grievances.

- When employees are feeling isolated and unconnected to the work group.

- When employees perceive that their strengths and backgrounds are not valued for the unique contribution they can make.

- When complaints are received about the behavior of patients and families.

If seeing these symptoms confirms the need for training, what can the organization expect as a result?

The benefits of training. When we discuss the benefits of training, we assume that the training itself is high caliber even though we know that that is not always the reality. A well-conducted, effective training session can enable employees to learn things about themselves that they did not know before. It can allow participants to engage in dialogue and explore complex issues that really have no right and wrong answers. It can also build understanding that helps employees to establish rapport that will help them when times get tough.

The limits of training. The biggest limit of training is the load it is expected to carry. Organizations are willing to bring executives together for two hours and employees together for a half or whole day, and at the end of these sessions they expect newly enlightened employees who through fresh insight and knowledge will change the organization and exhibit new individual behaviors. This view misses the fact that a lifetime of socialization does not change in a day. These expectations of training overlook what is being rewarded and what employees are being held accountable for day in and day out. Training can be valuable, but as a catalyst for change rather than as the vehicle that makes it happen.

The other limit of training is quality. Poor training creates far more problems than it can ever solve. Some organizations who have experienced bad training have taken years to get over it. The caveat here is: check out your trainers or consultants very carefully. Check their references, be very clear about what your training goals are, and watch them work. Work in partnership with the consultants you hire to make sure your specific needs are being met.

Remember, training is necessary for change, but not sufficient to make it happen. We suggest that having looked at the benefits and limits of training, and having assessed the symptoms you see in your workplace, you should focus the training content on two areas: increasing individual awareness and understanding, and developing competence around a set of managerial skills.

Training that focuses on individual awareness, attitudes, and beliefs. We always begin our awareness training with an overhead transparency that proclaims, "Diversity is an inside job." This is the essence of awareness training. It should help individuals to explore their own roots, cultural identity, and stereotypes. Specifically, three areas of training should be part of any organization's awareness segment:

- The organization's paradigm of diversity
- Culture as a key shaper of behavior
- Stereotypes and assumptions

Training that focuses on managerial skills. The focus of management training is skill building, with direct and immediate application. If such training is done well, a manager or supervisor should be able to take the skills and use them on the job the next day. Although any number of specific skills are appropriate, we suggest you pay attention to some of the following: performance review, conflict resolution, problem solving, conducting effective meetings, soliciting feedback, interviewing, hiring, and coaching. All of these skills have been taught for years in presumably monocultural environments. The idea behind teaching these managerial skills with a diversity bent is to add to the repertoire of managers' choices of behavior. They are not trading in one skill set for another, nor are they deleting skills. Rather, the goal is to expand effective managerial behaviors.

Measure and Evaluate

When all is said and done, does any of what your organization chooses to do around diversity make a difference? This is the time to go back to the criteria that were defined up front. The data can be measured in concrete statistics, such as retention and absenteeism figures, or in anecdotal data about patient satisfaction. If problems surfaced in focus group data, for example, it would be important to go back to the group and elicit follow-up data after an intervention was tried.

The issue of measurement and evaluation continues to be the most problematic because when people want hard numbers about the impact of a long-term initiative, it is impossible to isolate and quantify diversity training, changes in flex time, or same-sex partner benefits as reasons for increased commitment, greater productivity, or increased tenacity in problem solving. Testimonial data, while much easier to get, carries less weight with CFOs.

Allstate Insurance Company has been working on creating an inclusive organization for a very long time, and has found a clever way to evaluate and measure. The company annually administers an organizational audit of employee satisfaction that includes the question, "Have you had diversity training?" They then quantify a number of statistics for those who have had it and those who have not. Bingo! They have some of the proof they want. To date they have found that they do see a positive difference in a number of their indicators around satisfaction, problem solving, and conflict resolution.

All organizations involved in any diversity work are asking, "Does attention to diversity matter?" Answers are hard to come by. Most organizations are proceeding because they feel intuitively that it does, and they can use turnover figures, EEOC data, and other sources to confirm that intuition. But the area of measurement is still ripe for more work.

Follow-Up

Whatever initiatives are implemented, it is certain that modifications, refinements, and midcourse corrections will be required. Follow-up is the part of the process that really demonstrates accountability. Without it, efforts will be hollow and unachieved.

Organizational Barriers to Diversity

The process outlined in this chapter is comprehensive and doable, even though it is lengthy. The potential benefits to an organization are enormous. Considering the macro health care factors that are pushing toward a medical systems' full investment of time, energy, and resources in numerous change-related areas, and considering all that an organization can gain by going through the process, what possible obstacles could derail the initiative? Why might some executive staffs and organizations never even step up to the plate?

It is one thing to understand the three arenas for managing diversity discussed at the beginning of the chapter; it is something else altogether to manage those three arenas in an organization so that diversity becomes a recognizable asset that affects the bottom line. Serious barriers present real obstacles. The following eight barriers are among the most formidable stumbling blocks to a hospital's attempt to deal with diversity. They are the arguments we hear most frequently about why not to start this work in the first place. One of these may relate to your organization.

Cost of implementation. The noted economist Milton Friedman quipped that "there are no free lunches." His comment applies to health care organizations of the nineties. If a health care institution is serious about creating a culture that embraces diversity, what will it cost? Does an organization need bilingual software? Full-time translators? More training so employees can learn about the cultures they serve? What will be the gain from this investment? If all of this very necessary training takes place—and it is necessary if the diversity effort is going to be successful—who will be cranking out the work while staff is being trained? We can make a strong case for saying that the short-term cost may be high but the long-term benefits are worth it. With every health care dollar being microscopically scrutinized, getting a commitment of resources can be a major obstacle.

Fear of hiring underskilled, uneducated employees. In our work with numerous clients, the biggest issue in diversity hiring is the presumption that hiring women, people of color, and other segments of the population that fall under the diversity banner will mean sacrificing competence and quality. Common stereotypes hold that members of some groups are less educated and therefore less able to function in a work environment. These stereotypes do not necessarily have any validity. Recall the St. Francis experiment described in Chapter Seven. This hospital is hiring and training employees from the community so they can gain skills, and the results so far are positive. The big concern at St. Francis and other medical centers is, "If we make the investment, will the employees stay and will they be able to do the work?" Note also that health care institutions that hire from their respective communities will reap the rewards of goodwill engendered throughout the community.

Strong belief in a system that favors merit. There is a bias toward equal treatment in this country that in itself is commendable. What makes this otherwise admirable attitude a barrier toward diversity, however, can be found in the subtle aphorism we have been raised on, the one that advocates the best *man* for the job. In the United States, not only has the best, or *only*, person for a job historically been a man, but it has also been a white man. It is not uncommon for hospitals, medical centers, and HMOs to be full of diversity—at lower levels. There is plenty of diversity among the housekeeping, cafeteria, nursing, and lab technician staff. Organizations have been dragged, kicking and screaming, toward affirmative action as a way to level the playing field, but the perception still exists that any affirmative action candidate is chosen to fill a slot, not because she may happen to be the best candidate for the job. Our socialization over the years is so strong and our biases so subtle that women or persons of color are not commonly considered the best person for the job.

Annoyance at reverse discrimination. Reverse discrimination raises the hackles of those fair play advocates who say that it does not help to end discrimination of one group at the expense of another. So long as one person's gain is perceived to be someone else's loss, fears of reverse discrimination will provide very strong resistance to diversity. In interviewing people about their recruitment practices, organizations that were effectively dealing with diversity looked for employees from very diverse backgrounds. Sometimes, however, the applicant pool did not allow them to be as diverse as they would have liked. They did not sacrifice quality, but what they did do, when they did find a number of excellent candidates from different groups, was take into consideration the ethnic makeup of their employee base.

Perception that there has been a lot of progress. In the eyes of some, any progress that exists is proof that the system, health care or otherwise, is opening up. If it opens at a snail's pace, so what? The thought goes something like this: women, people of color, the differently abled, the older worker, and whoever is not part of the dominant group should all appreciate the crack in the door. Be satisfied with the progress you have made, is the implied message. It is generally true in hospitals across the board that female employees often feel a need to assert themselves in dealing with male physicians, yet they still rarely do so. They feel as though their voices are not heard, that respect is not given, and that their dignity is diminished. These feelings are expensive. Our view is that somewhere between the slow evolution that some advocate and the revolution that others want is a median point that would serve the American health care industry well. But as long as there is an attitude that "things are much better, what more do you want?" we will cheat organizations of talent and create a disenfranchisement that will only be harmful down the road.

Diversity not seen as a top-priority issue. In a long list of organizational priorities, diversity may not be seen as crucial or bottom-line. The organizational complaint mill usually works overtime when any change occurs, but expect it to work longer and harder when it comes to diversity. The psychological adaptations required of employees in the workforce today are numerous and demanding. Mergers and downsizing are already problematic, and this is just one more issue heaped on others that make people dissatisfied. The beef will be, "If it isn't crucial,"—and some think embracing a more open and diverse culture is not—"then why mess with it? It only saps energy from the really important issues at hand."

Need to dismantle the existing systems to accommodate diversity. The sheer weight of rethinking or changing existing systems is frightening to many people. Some fear the changes because of what they perceive they will lose. If, for example, the selection process or reward structure or performance review system is changed to create a more inclusive environment, what will that mean to the many employees in your organization? We suspect that some people will be helped while others may be hurt. There is a perception by employees that in any transaction that creates a new system based on diversity issues, they will lose opportunity, power, and resources. If you are charged with the task of modifying the existing systems, it will take a lot of work to develop a plan and get employees to buy into it. Part of the buy-in involves including benefits for everyone. If you are charged with implementing the new system, it means learning and teaching new methods of operation to others and then setting up a feedback system. And if you are an employee affected by these changes, you probably do not know what it will mean, and that might be the scariest position of all.

Inertia. Your organization is analogous to a human system whose primary function is to sustain and perpetuate itself. Any outside intervention is viewed as threatening, so the system closes to protect itself from intrusion. The result? Sheer inertia will keep the system moving on its steady course; hence, organizational and personal responses to change almost guarantee that reversing or changing direction will not happen easily.

When all is said and done, making substantive changes is an arduous task. Faint-of-heart organizations may offer a little diversity awareness training or pass out diversity calendars to foster sensitivity, but the timid will not, and should not, embark on the road of real cultural change. Fixing systems so that they work better for everyone is a demanding, comprehensive job that offers little gratitude, and some complaints and dislocation along the way. But for organizations that embark on the path and achieve success, life is never the same. Success is not only defined by achieving specific criteria, it is also defined by the passion, commitment, and energy of people working together to achieve something great. We will not romanticize the journey. It is fraught with land mines and potholes and all manner of obstacles. But accomplishment is meaningful, revenue enhancing, rewarding, and rejuvenating. It is the trip of a lifetime for those willing to make the journey.

9

Creative Organizational Problem Solving

Surging costs, decreased reimbursements, multiple languages, staff reductions and higher patient acuity are only a few of the changes that put pressure on health care providers to do more with less. For institutions, this national health care crisis translates into multiple challenges. Providing high quality care in an increasingly diverse environment is today's reality, and organizations in the forefront have taken the bull by the horns in devising some creative methods for meeting these challenges. This chapter presents some examples of how four health care organizations did just that.

Demographics-Driven Marketing

Little Company of Mary, a respected hospital in Torrance, California, began to notice some changes in its patient population in the 1980s. More and more Japanese-speaking patients were coming to the hospital, especially pregnant women for childbirth. The hospital was also getting frequent calls from Japanese men seeking physical examinations. Staff politely explained that the institution did not do physicals and that the patient would need to arrange with his regular physician for such an exam. Luckily for the hospital, one Japanese business leader in the community saw what was happening and came to talk to the hospital's CEO and explain what he saw as an unmet need. Kurt Miyamoto, Japanese expatriate working in the United States and then vice president of the Japan Business Association of Southern California, South Bay Chapter, had some very important information to share.

The South Bay area surrounding the hospital was home to more than 250 Japanese companies, such as Toyota, Nissan, and Honda, operating in the United States. These firms employed many executives who were sent from Japan to U.S. locations on three- to five-year assignments and who were living with their families in communities in the hospital's service area. What Little Company of Mary did not know but soon learned was that Japanese firms place a great deal of emphasis on prevention in health care. Because of that emphasis, they require their executives to have complete physical exams annually. For the past thirty-five years this annual checkup for executives has been a standard business practice in Japan and the service is offered by most hospitals there. Not only was it natural for the Japanese executives to expect a similar service in the United States but they also preferred the hospital-based approach because they felt that the coordination of complex tests and the analysis of results could be done better by a hospital than by individual physicians.

When Little Company of Mary Hospital realized that it had been presented with a golden opportunity, it responded by creating the Ningen Dock program. Named after the Human Dry Dock, a Japanese annual executive physical, the program provides this desired but previously unavailable service. To begin with, seven then finally nine Japanese-speaking physicians were recruited, and the most sophisticated software and computer system for this program was obtained from Japan. A full-time Japanese interpreter was hired. In addition, Japanese-speaking nurses and a bilingual clerk were hired. The hospital then held meetings to explain the Ningen Dock program to physicians and staff, discussing the reasons for the program and its purpose. All areas of the hospital were included in these meetings because the program required the cooperation and coordination of departments across the hospital, from admitting, lab, and radiology to dietary. In addition, Japanese classes were given to staff so they could learn a little of the language and culture. Bilingual signs and brochures were posted in the hospital and at the free-standing clinic where the Ningen Dock program resides.

Beyond getting employees to commit to the program, the hospital faced another challenge. Additional staff were required, yet at the beginning the program did not have enough patients to generate the money to pay for them. Seeing clearly that the program would run in the red during the start-up phase, the hospital took the risk of footing the start-up costs and hired the necessary staff anyway.

Word of mouth in the small, tightly knit Japanese expatriate community in the South Bay quickly spread the news about Ningen Dock. Information about services and prices passed along the grapevine. Statistics show that the majority of Japanese patients are referred by colleagues, associates, and friends. The initial goal of the program, that Little Company of Mary would be the hospital of first choice among Japanese, was soon achieved.

The program superseded its own goals, however. Because of the excellent quality of care they felt they had received at the hospital, seven Japanese executives volunteered to raise funds for the hospital's Capital Campaign 2000. Though this kind of volunteer fundraising activity is virtually unknown in Japan, these businessmen have already collected $240,000 in donations for the hospital. Much of this process has been assisted by Kurt Miyamoto, who has been working with Little Company of Mary and this program for the last seven years and now serves as the executive advisor to the Japanese program.

Though the Ningen Dock program functions in a stand-alone clinic, its users and their families have health care needs that go beyond the annual executive checkup. The hospital has responded to these needs as well. Japanese-speaking employees work on various floors and assist and translate on the obstetrics and gynecology floor. Food services has expanded its menu to include Japanese dietary preferences such as rice, miso soup, and green tea.

"Providing Japanese patients with a level of comfort and peace of mind makes the Ningen Dock program very special," according to Yoko Cummings, supervisor of the program. An important part of this service is the Japanese Helpline. "When patients go to the hospital in Japan, they receive one bill that includes all hospital services. Here, Japanese patients are often confused by the numerous bills they receive. They also need help with the translation and interpretation, so they call the Helpline," says Kiyo Noto, Japanese interpreter and a big part of the program. The Helpline, in operation since 1989, provides a physician referral service; helps with admission, translation and interpretation, maternity tours, company tours, and clarification of insurance and billing; and assists with patient treatment and emergency room visits.

Clearly Kiyo's work goes beyond merely interpreting. In addition to visiting each Japanese patient every day, Kiyo gives good service a new definition by doing such things as conducting maternity tours on weekends by patient request so that husbands who work Monday through Saturday can accompany their wives. When Japanese patients come to the emergency room, Kiyo meets them there, then contacts other departments to smooth the way. "When I help these Japanese patients in the hospital, I offer them my support, listen to their stories, and speak to them in Japanese. Having someone who can understand them is both encouraging and comforting."

As testimony to the program's success, almost 12 percent of the patients at Little Company of Mary are Japanese and more than nine hundred executives and their spouses have participated in the program.

Kaiser Permanente Southern California Mentoring and Coaching

The need to develop people inside the organization is an issue that crosses industries, geography, and functional levels. Mentoring and coaching are among the traditional ways organizations take their underrepresented employees and groom them for increased responsibility and expansion of their skill sets and job descriptions.

Although there are many vehicles and strategies for coaching and mentoring, the data on these two strategies have so far yielded mixed results. However, Kaiser Permanente, Southern California, has achieved some very clear gains. For that reason, we are sharing their process.

In 1991, Kaiser Permanente Southern California, headquartered in Pasadena, originated a way to develop minorities and women in management through a mentoring project. In the years 1991–1995 the program had five goals that were met and remained in effect into 1996. These goals were

- Transmitting organizational goals and improving organizational climate
- Transferring critical skills and knowledge
- Developing future leaders
- Demonstrating the value of the individual employee
- Fostering the development of minority managers

Each year from 1991 on, some new process or feature was implemented. What made the 1996 experience such a unique one was the addition of group mentoring, a simultaneous alternative to the one-on-one mentoring. The group structure provided the opportunity for two to four protégés to work with one mentor. A big plus in this process was the peer learning. Participants also received instruction, role modeling, and coaching by the mentor. Because the design involved cross-functional, cross-departmental grouping, protégés had the opportunity to see a wide swath of the organization, and to use the protégé group as a safe harbor in which to discuss or look for solutions to difficult problems.

The 1996 mentors represented a variety of high-level positions at Kaiser. Two were hospital administrators, one was a regional medical director, and several were assistant medical and hospital group administrators. There were two medical group administrators, three pharmacy chiefs, and several human resource administrators.

The protégés were also drawn from a wide variety of backgrounds throughout the organization. Among the participants being mentored were managers from housekeeping, pharmacy, human resources, public affairs, and assorted medical departments. Of the nineteen protégés, fifteen were women and four were men. Eight were African American, eight were Caucasian, two were Latino, and one was Asian. Kaiser specifically tells participants, in a move designed to clarify expectations, that the objective of the mentoring program is not to achieve promotions. Nevertheless, eight of the protégés did receive promotions in the 1996 mentoring program year.

Beyond the gender, racial, and ethnic composition, those who designed the program wanted broad diversity representation. With that goal in mind, participants were chosen from different functional levels and different geographic locations. In addition, they had different areas of job focus so they could learn from one another. The program was designed to deepen protégé's understanding of different jobs and skills important to the organization.

Feedback was obtained through a midyear progress report of evaluations, phone interviews, closing session activities, and a final e-mail questionnaire. Anecdotal remarks by participants, both mentors and protégés, indicate that the group mentoring structure provided plentiful food for thought. The following quotes are taken from the evaluation data:

> "I found the sharing during our group discussion very productive. . . . (It) gave me lots of insights, examples I could practice in my job environment."

> "The thing that worked best for me was the group process itself. If I was having a tough time with a particular problem, others in the group who had experienced similar problems would assist me with problem solving."

The mentor's perspective was that the group allows people to feed off one another and in so doing improves the quality of the discussion.

The group mentoring process, difficult to coordinate due to the numerous schedules of very busy people, does present a real challenge. Participants have to work hard to get together. Sometimes life and other responsibilities get in the way and energy sags. One of Kaiser's original reasons for doing group mentoring was that it offered a way to groom and coach more people than if the organization used only labor-intensive one-on-one relationships. While both one-on-one and group mentoring yielded results, the group structure had the advantage of protégés functioning as peer tutors. In addition to providing good cross-pollination for ideas and a safe place to discuss problems, the group was also a means to get practical feedback in a safe environment.

Among the lessons learned from the mentoring program were that some mentors required more clearly defined roles than others. Feedback indicates that the mentoring resulted in people, particularly protégés, recommitting to the organization.

Among the challenges that Kaiser faces is maintaining momentum. This is difficult to do, particularly in a group setting, in which multiple schedules need to be coordinated. There is no easy answer to this dilemma. The time issue raises another, related problem: mentors chafe at the extra work involved. Furthermore, some do not see how they can be helpful if protégés have a different career field. Nevertheless, participating Kaiser personnel indicate that they learn a great deal individually and collectively.

Another innovative approach to developing managers at Kaiser is through specially trained "diversity coaches." This new program is aimed at training those staff members, such as human resource consultants and Employee Assistance Program professionals, to whom managers come when they have problems with employees. Training enables them to give one-on-one coaching to help managers deal with diversity-related challenges. Delivering this coaching help on a "just in time" basis at the request of the manager taps into a fundamental concept of adult learning motivation, which is that adults are at their best as learners when they have an immediate and clearly defined need and use for the learning. The Kaiser diversity coach program utilizes a one-and-a-half-day training design focusing on three main content areas: the influence of culture on workplace interactions, how to identify and question assumptions made about others' behavior, and conflict resolution.

Because physicians are measured on their ability to interact positively with patients, it was strongly felt that Kaiser had a responsibility to provide them with tools to improve their skills in this arena as well. The video coaching program was created to fill this need. Physicians volunteer to come and be videotaped "interfacing with" an actor who plays the role of a patient in a simulated visit. Actors from different cultural groups experienced at portraying patients from various backgrounds and orientations create a sense of reality in the simulated visits. The tape is then reviewed by two coaches and the physician. Coaches give feedback and facilitate observations and understanding gained from the taped simulations. The power of the process is in the immediacy and relevance of the feedback. Eighty-five percent of physicians reported that they learned something from the coaching and that it was helpful. The video coaching program offers a unique opportunity for physicians to practice important patient interaction skills.

Another method of coaching physicians is through a workshop that deals specifically with interactions between physicians and patients of diverse cultural backgrounds. Topics such as how to most effectively conduct an interpreted medical encounter, what potential cultural barriers might prevent patient adherence to a treatment regimen, and the significance of traditional or folk medical beliefs are covered. The Kaiser Permanente National Diversity Council developed handbooks on the health beliefs and epidemiology of specific patient populations to support this effort.

Providing Health Care to the Underserved: A Revolutionary Plan

The poor, elderly, and disabled are among the most critically underserved populations in health care. Although many attempts have been made to deal with this gaping hole in the medical system, perhaps none is as far-reaching and strategic as LA Care Health Plan. Formed by the State Department of Health Services to help Medi-Cal services make the transition from fee-for-service to managed care, this fundamentally new arrangement attempts to solve the kinds of problems that prevent poor, elderly, and other underserved patients from getting adequate care, as well as to deliver high-quality care in a cost-effective way.

LA Care Health Plan contracts with several HMOs, including Blue Cross of California Health Plans, Care 1st Health Plan, Maxicare of California, Tower Health, United Health Plan, LA County Community Health Plan, and Kaiser Foundation Health Plan. The object of the managed care program is not just to save money for the state; it is also to improve the health of the most vulnerable populations: children living in poverty, refugees, the elderly, mothers with dependent children, and those with disabilities. Through this program, these populations are educated and empowered to develop a relationship with a primary care provider and create a "medical home," a health care base for each patient. This provider, generally located within five to ten miles of the patient, has an obligation to see the patient for an initial health assessment within 120 days of enrollment so that a relationship can begin. The patient then has a doctor to call in an emergency rather than using the emergency room, and has a physician who takes an interest in preventive care and helping the patient maintain wellness. Members who traditionally only went to a doctor when they became seriously ill are offered a more proactive approach to health.

LA Care's mission statement is, "To ensure the provision of culturally sensitive and linguistically competent quality health care services to the Medi-Cal population in Los Angeles County through our health partners to promote health and disease prevention, to continuously improve the knowledge and effectiveness of our provider community, and to assist in the provision of the same quality of services for the vulnerable populations."

As part of its strategy to provide culturally sensitive and lin-guistically competent care, LA Care recruits health care providers who can communicate with members in their language of choice. Further, the plan coordinates the distribution of information to and the education of members in nine languages. In addition to English and a TDD phone line for the hearing impaired, outreach and help are provided in Spanish, Cambodian, Cantonese, Farsi, Hmong, Lao, Russian, and Vietnamese. LA Care's Education department includes staff who are fluent in these languages and have knowledge of the culture and health care needs of these ethnic groups. These educators work with community members, training them to be moderators using an educational video in each of the languages that explains the changes in Medi-Cal and the options available to members in choosing a plan that will meet their needs.

A critical part of the plan is the empowerment of state assis-tance recipients to take an active role in their own health care deci-sions. This is accomplished through education about the choices and benefits involved in the various options, the HMO plans, and the old fee-for-service system that is being phased out. Empower-ment at a more strategic level is also stimulated through regional community advisory conferences, committees made up of represen-tatives of actual beneficiaries, and health plan members, as well as providers and advocates who have input into state health care pol-icymaking.

Educators and community outreach staff have found creative ways to overcome some of the predictable as well as the surprising obstacles to community involvement. When the first meetings, set at hospital sites, were poorly attended, staff set about finding more comfortable, consumer- and beneficiary-friendly locations. United Way centers and Boys and Girls Clubs, for example, were often more familiar than hospitals to community members, and closer to bus routes. Educators and community outreach staff learned that language was not the only barrier to communication. Hispanic staff members advised them that the fun icebreakers planned to get everyone involved at meetings were intimidating and would have a negative effect on participation among many in that population. Staff also found that with some Latina members who were less vocal and assertive in meetings, establishing individual relationships and asking quietly for input got better results.

LA Care staff have been active in recruiting not only members but also their target group's providers. Primary care physicians who have traditionally treated many Medi-Cal patients may be independent practitioners who are not members of any of LA Care's partner plans, so staff work to get them included through a plan that allows patients to continue getting care from their trusted, long-time caregivers. Other providers, such as midwives, are also targeted with programs to help raise the quality of education and increase credentialing of those whose caseload has been made up of at least 15 percent Medi-Cal patients.

With its emphasis on preventive care, empowerment, and education of vulnerable and historically underserved populations, LA Care offers an approach that may provide new lessons for other health care organizations facing similar challenges.

A Systemic Commitment to Caring for the Underserved

Yakima County is located in the South-central portion of Washington state. It is the second largest county in area and the seventh largest county in population in the state. The largest land holdings are the federally reserved trust lands of the Yakima Indian Reservation, 1.1 million acres, or 40 percent of the county. Between the various tribes and the state and federal government, almost 73 percent of the land is spoken for. The biggest industry in the county by far is agriculture, with apples being Yakima's main claim to agricultural fame. While agriculture can be a very lucrative industry, not all residents seem to share equally in the wealth. A full 31 percent of households make less than $15,000 annually. In 1994, of the 110,000 adults in the county, a little over 90,000 were employed, leaving approximately 20,000 unemployed.

There have been interesting shifts in the population. As of 1995, the white population was a little more than 122,000; the Hispanic population, growing rapidly, was 68,000. The Native American population was approximately 8,800, with the number of Asians slightly edging out the number of blacks, 2,178 to 2,067. Hispanics and Native Americans are quite young, with a large number of very young children and young adults in their child-bearing years, indicating continued rapid growth in these groups.

It is in the middle of this rural area that Sisters of Providence Health System has its Central Washington Service Area and that the communities of Toppenish and Yakima have facilities that care for and attend to the local populations previously mentioned. SPHS in Central Washington, even by the standards of this farsighted organization, is tenacious about operationalizing diversity throughout the Yakima and Toppenish facilities and in the clinics as well. To give a sense of the company's commitment and desire to make diversity a way of life throughout the organization, we share some attitudes, actions, and initiatives at the administrative, physician, diversity council, and managerial levels. We also acknowledge a remarkable community outreach program called Team Apple. Each of these groups makes a significant contribution to serving its diverse and mostly poor population in the Central Washington Service Area.

Administrators

Steve Burdick, operations administrator of Providence Toppenish, and Barbara Hood, CEO of the Service Area, described the ways in which hospital staff have become sensitive to the various employee populations, and how important it is to honor the uniqueness of the various cultures. As an example, Steve described the Family Maternity Center for Native Americans. An obstetrics patient who is Native American may have different needs for privacy and beliefs about body fluid replacement than a non–Native American. Members of the Tribal Council met with SPHS nurse managers about these and other concerns. As a result of receiving culturally relevant information from the Tribal Council, SPHS conducted training to heighten staff sensitivities.

Burdick's predecessor led a strong effort to meet the needs of this group, but he continues the effort in a direct but not overly aggressive way. He sees his job as translating or interpreting the mission and values into tangible expectations for the folks involved. Toward that end, SPHS's Toppenish facility has created a Native American Spiritual Center, a place for Native Americans to pray, celebrate rituals, and be faithful to the spiritual ways that facilitate healing and harmony that are always part of a health care process. Steve has also talked about paying attention to the dietary needs of different populations. The facility serves Indian tacos on rye bread because these gestures are necessary as symbolic indicators of inclusion. The more substantive changes Steve is working toward include developing a workforce that more closely resembles the patient population of the Toppenish facility. He believes that Toppenish has the most reflective minority makeup of staff to community of anyplace in the system, but it is not good enough, particularly among physicians and in the areas of technical expertise. Steve mentioned an existing program that he is proud of, one that could benefit from even more development. It offers educational subsidies for both the Native American and the Hispanic populations. The youth, kids from high school and community college, have done summer residences in which they rotate internships in health care. It is a good way to expose these young people to the profession and to groom them to learn a job and stay in the community.

Barbara Hood wants to model the behavior she seeks from staff. She has no time or patience for discrimination, and if she hears comments or language that violate tenets of respect, she calls people on it and tells them that their language is unacceptable. When she gets accused of driving thoughts or comments underground, that is fine with her. She wants certain language and behaviors to be recognized as unacceptable, and if people cannot understand and abide by certain norms, she respectfully indicates that her organization is not the place for them.

Barbara is strategic in getting support and building relationships. When she came to the area, the hospital was losing a lot of money. She asked the Sisters of Providence to match any investment she could raise. They did, and a new medical building is being built and financed.

The Physicians

Toppenish is blessed to have many excellent and caring physicians. One of them, David Cassidy, is a family physician who serves a mostly Hispanic population. Cassidy and his colleagues try to know the whole patient and understand lifestyle, stress, and other variables that might have an impact on illness or disease. They say that the biggest changes regarding diversity have come with a new administration. The previous administrator had little interest in this issue, but recently, one employee was fired because of the way she treated Hispanics. This woman, who was Native American and probably no novice to ridicule and prejudice herself, was openly hostile, patronizing, and demeaning to patients of Hispanic origin. For this she was let go.

When administrators hold staff accountable, it creates a much more supportive climate for doctors trying to work with poor, less educated populations. Some of the challenge comes from being in a rural community where it is difficult to find highly trained staff in general, much less bilingual staff. But there is a sense that the sisters have a clear and compassionate mission, and for these physicians the administration and the dedication of the medical staff create a very good partnership, and some very lucky patients.

The Diversity Council

SPHS convened a diversity council, which is responsible for shepherding the initiative throughout the system. The council's view was a balanced one. The members loved the training, they believe that diversity initiatives, which have helped both internal and external populations, are critically important. They already see the results of the training in the increase in sensitivity as staff members interact with patients and families.

But the council's big sadness is that they weigh the potential gains of long-term diversity initiatives against the lack of resources to make change happen. There is often insufficient funding and time to do what all the people want to do. At the most fundamental level, lack of time is a killer. Council meetings fall through the cracks. There are scheduling problems, and it is hard to get a good meeting time for everyone, so momentum dips.

Council members have one thing in common with the managers. Both groups feel that attention to diversity is essential and offers clear benefits; however, they acknowledge that the lack of financial resources is a stumbling block, particularly in the area of funding for translators. The light at the end of the tunnel is in the positive attitude toward diversity and the very real need that people see to devote time and attention to diversity-related issues.

Team Apple

The most impressive manifestation of diversity work in Toppenish takes place in a community health alliance called Team Apple. It is a one-year-old organization that significantly affects the lives of previously underserved populations who were afraid of and distant from traditional health care organizations. The team consists of a unique group of professionals. Kathy Bambrick, a team leader from Team Apple, is a registered dietitian who has served as coordinator and manager of the child health program and now serves as coordinator for the Healthy Communities Alliance. Dee Nunez was born in Mexico, came to SPHS in 1989 to do volunteer work, and continues to migrate seasonally back and forth between Mexico and Washington. Mary Pellicier is a medical director, a family practice physician who now functions full-time in an administrative role.

Colleen Kaluzny, who has a master's degree in family counseling, designs programs that try to instill better parenting skills. Naomi Ojctus is stationed at a local parish. She works to build trust and establish relationships. She also does outreach, trying to bring health care access to a needy population. Among these women are many years of experience in their fields, competence, dedication, and a passion to accomplish their mission of serving this community.

Team Apple started out teaching traditional obstetrics classes in a hospital, but only a few people would sign up and, for a variety of reasons, none would show up. Physicians kept wanting more classes, but the services being offered were not being utilized. The organization could not justify starting a much-needed parenting program when no one would even come to classes on prenatal care and child birth. This dilemma became the catalyst for the birth of Healthy Communities Alliance and the other entities that now exist. The organization knew that people wanted the education in the most basic skills, like brushing teeth, but they would not show up for reasons unique to each community. The traditional assessment approach to health care and social services did not work. Instead, Team Apple developed a partnership with the community residents that resulted in the following:

• Naomi, who is a Sister of Providence, a nurse, and a spiritual leader, found out that one family in the community needed insurance, so she found a way to sell it because they wanted it and needed it. In the process she was building trust, and the hope that they would go to the clinic for other needs as well.

• A health professional gave basic health and hygiene tips, which resulted in a group of Hispanic women in Wapato setting up exercise classes several days a week. They eliminated their depression and increased their self-esteem. Ultimately they organized an enchilada and baked goods sale to raise money to buy exercise outfits. This is preventive health care in action. Some of these women are now talking about becoming aerobics instructors and becoming licensed.

- A staff member worked with a Spanish parenting group that meets once a month. Twenty-five parents were organizing day care, planning graduation, and figuring out how to give awards to children. They had a raffle for a live pig, had fun, raised money, and accomplished business.

- A Team Apple staffer gave empowerment classes to parents, providing them with basic hands-on information and demonstrating skill building, teeth brushing, and child development.

- Colleen helped a family whose teenage daughter had a lump in her breast get another opinion from a surgeon who was willing to do the procedure for free. The surgeon was 99 percent sure that the tumor was benign. This surgeon helped the family get their sense of control back and achieve both financial and emotional relief.

- Dee set up discussions in a local restaurant on the night it was closed so that women could come together, share experiences, and offer one another support. When one member's husband did not want her to go, Dee interceded by going to see him, explaining the reasons his wife should attend the meetings and assuring him in ways he could understand that her participation was no reflection on him. His image and reputation were safe.

How did all of these very good things happen? Two answers explain the ability of these providers to be of such service. The first answer is their strategic thinking skills. Stationing Naomi in a church, for example, where Mexicans go on a regular basis, is one example of how clever these service providers are. If you are trying to reach the community, you go where it is. Team Apple staff are also willing to meet the potential patients where they are educationally and emotionally, rather than using only the traditional model of diagnosing an illness and treating it. For the group of women who organize and run the programs, health is not merely an absence of disease. It is an optimum state of physical, mental, social, and spiritual wholeness or wellness. Housing is a health issue. Illiteracy is a health issue. The Community Alliance likes to help people help themselves in whatever areas of their lives are not working.

The other element that makes the Community Health Alliance special is its philosophy. It is seen and designed to be a real partnership so that the administrators and caregivers get their cues from the people they serve.

In all the case studies we have presented here, we wanted you to get a glimpse of the possibilities, but also of the realities. None of these organizations is living in paradise. They are all rooted in very complex realities. Nevertheless, in spite of all the obstacles and sticking points, they have made good things happen, and you can too with equal tenacity, commitment, and passion.

Resources

Books About Diversity in Health Care

Decalmer, P., and Glendinning, F. (eds.). *The Mistreatment of Elderly People*. Thousand Oaks, Calif.: Sage, 1993. This book discusses elder abuse, including the clinical and legal implications as well as the issues for nurses and physicians.

Galanti, G.-A. *Caring for Patients from Different Cultures: Case Studies from American Hospitals*. Philadelphia: University of Pennsylvania Press, 1991. This pertinent book written by a professor of nursing and anthropology describes more than 135 actual culture conflicts that have occurred in American hospitals. Its purpose is to help health care professionals understand the cultural dimensions of problems that occur between staff and patients and their families. The book also contains an extensive bibliography for those desiring more specific information.

Gropper, R. C. *Culture and the Clinical Encounter: An Intercultural Sensitizer for the Health Professions*. Yarmouth, Maine: Intercultural Press, 1996. Through the use of critical incidents, the author, a medical anthropologist, gives western-trained health care providers insightful examples of the health care beliefs and practices of many cultures. Each incident presents a cross-cultural problem in a clinical context, for which the reader must choose the best of four possible explanations. The choices are then explained, with reasons given for why a choice is or is not the best course of action.

Helman, C. G. *Culture, Health and Illness*. Oxford: Butterworth-Heine-mann, 1994. This medical anthropology work provides in-depth explo-ration of the ways in which different cultural, social, and ethnic groups explain the cause of illness, the kinds of treatments they believe in, and the healers they prefer. Chapters include topics such as gender and repro-duction, doctor-patient interaction, and cultural definitions of anatomy and physiology.

Kao, H.S.R., and Durganand, S. (eds.). *Asian Perspectives on Psychology*. Thousand Oaks, Calif.: Sage, 1996. This collection of articles by experts from different Asian countries presents perspectives on socialization, development, emotion, personality, and approaches to health.

Kaslow, D. R., and Salett, E. P. (eds.). *Crossing Cultures in Mental Health*. Washington, D.C.: Sietar International, 1989. Through a series of arti-cles, this book offers insight and suggestions for improving cross-cultural communication, especially with regard to immigrant and refugee popula-tions. Both general and culture-specific information is given.

Lorber, J. *Gender and the Social Construction of Illness*. Thousand Oaks, Calif.: Sage, 1997. In this book, the author brings a feminist perspective to examining the interface between gender and Western medicine. Chap-ters include "The Doctor Knows Best: Gender and the Medical Encounter" and "If a Situation is Defined as Real: Premenstrual Syndrome and Menopause."

The National Coalition of Hispanic Health and Human Services Orga-nizations, *Delivering Preventive Health Care to Hispanics: A Manual for Providers*. Washington, D.C.: The National Coalition of Hispanic Health and Human Services Organizations, 1990. This rich resource in notebook form contains critical information about providing health care to His-panics. Chapters include information on beliefs and practices, strategies for effective patient provider interaction, community education, and spe-cific health problems.

Salimbene, S., and Graczykowski, J. W. *What Language Does Your Patient Hurt In? A Health Practitioner's Guide to Treating Patients from Other Cul-tures*. Amherst, Mass.: Amherst Educational Publishing, 1998. This user-friendly guide addresses the practical issues involved in the interaction between culture and health care. Both fundamental information about general cultural influences on medical care and specific information about the major culture and language groups in the United States are provided.

Secundy, M. G., and Nixon, L. L. *Trials, Tribulations and Celebrations: African-American Perspectives on Health, Illness, Aging and Loss.* Yarmouth, Maine: Intercultural Press, 1992. This collection of short stories, narratives, and poems explores aspects of the life cycle from an African American perspective. It is especially helpful for health care providers who provide services in a multicultural society.

Waxler-Morrison, N., Anderson, J., and Richardson, E. (eds.). *Cross Cultural Caring: A Handbook for Health Professionals.* Vancouver, B.C.: University of British Columbia Press, 1990. This handbook provides information on recent immigrant groups in Western Canada, such as Vietnamese, Chinese, Japanese, West Indians, and Iranians. Each chapter, written by a health care professional from that culture, focuses on the health care beliefs and practices as well as on the social context of each group.

Wiseman, R. L. (ed.). *Intercultural Communication Theory.* Thousand Oaks, Calif.: Sage, 1995. This series of scholarly papers on intercultural communication includes a pertinent chapter on cultural differences that have an impact on health care communication, giving culture-specific examples.

General Books About Diversity

Allport, G. W. *The Nature of Prejudice.* Reading, Mass.: Addison-Wesley, 1988. This classic study of the roots of discrimination, originally published in 1954, offers important information, understanding, and insights about dealing with prejudice and stereotyping.

Arredondo, P. *Successful Diversity Management Initiatives: A Blueprint for Planning and Implementation.* Thousand Oaks, Calif.: Sage, 1996. This recent addition to the field presents specific steps to plan, direct, and guide organizations through diversity implementation, giving vignettes based on organizational experiences.

Baytos, L. M. *Designing and Implementing Successful Diversity Programs*. Englewood Cliffs, N.J.: Prentice Hall, 1995. This thorough how-to manual provides practical guidance and tools to assist practitioners charged with implementing diversity. Organizational examples as well as checklists and assessments are provided.

Brown, C. D., Snedeker, C. C., and Sykes, B. D. *Conflict and Diversity*. Cresskill, N.J.: Hampton Press, 1997. This book presents chapters, all by outstanding communication and diversity management experts, that address different facets of workplace conflict. It offers theoretical approaches, research, and case studies to help the reader understand diversity-related barriers, as well as tools to deal with them.

Gardenswartz, L., and Rowe, A. *Managing Diversity: A Complete Desk Reference and Planning Guide*. Burr Ridge, Ill.: Irwin, 1993. This comprehensive guide that includes both conceptual information and practical techniques gives a myriad of strategies and activities for managing diversity. More than eighty worksheets, checklists, and charts are provided for use by managers, trainers, consultants, and human resource professionals.

Gudykunst, W. B. *Bridging Differences: Effective Intergroup Communication*. Thousand Oaks, Calif.: Sage, 1991. This book explains the process underlying communication between people of different groups and presents principles for building community with people from diverse backgrounds.

Gudykunst, W. B., Stewart, L. P., and Ting-Toomey, S. (eds.). *Communication, Culture, and Organizational Processes*. Thousand Oaks, Calif.: Sage, 1985. This collection of articles weaves theoretical issues with practical, organizational concerns such as conflict, negotiation, and decision making in multicultural settings.

Hall, E. T. *Beyond Culture*. Garden City, New York: Anchor Books, 1989. This foundation piece on cross-cultural communication analyzes in depth the culturally determined yet unconscious attitudes that mold our thoughts, feelings, communication, and behavior. It continues from the author's earlier books *The Silent Language* and *The Hidden Dimension* to discuss the covert cultural influences that affect cross-cultural encounters.

Hall, E. T. *The Hidden Dimension*. New York: Anchor Books, 1969. This book explains proxemics, the ways humans use space in public and in private. It provides insights about how this aspect of culture affects personal and business relations and cross-cultural interactions as well as architecture and urban planning.

Hall, E. T. *The Silent Language*. New York: Anchor Books, 1973. Information about the cultural aspects of communication is put forth in this fundamental work. The author explains how dimensions such as time and space communicate beyond words.

Harris, P. R., and Moran, R. T. *Managing Cultural Differences: High-Performance Strategies for Today's Global Manager*. Houston: Gulf, 1987. This business-oriented text on diversity gives a comprehensive treatment of the cultural differences affecting business, focusing more on international than on domestic intercultural issues. It includes questionnaires, surveys, and resources.

Hayles, R., and Russell, A. M. *The Diversity Directive: Why Some Initiatives Fail and What to Do About It*. Burr Ridge, Ill.: Irwin, 1997. Drawing on extensive corporate experience, the authors outline the steps necessary for implementing effective diversity initiatives.

Herbert, P. H. *The Color of Words: An Encyclopaedic Dictionary of Ethnic Bias in the United States*. Yarmouth, Maine: Intercultural Press, 1997. This thought-provoking book explains the power of language and how it is used to express bias and hatred toward "others." More than 850 words, expressions, and phrases that carry bias are explained.

Hofstede, G. *Cultures and Organizations: Software of the Mind*. New York: McGraw-Hill, 1991. In this work the author shows that effective intercultural cooperation is possible and explains under what circumstances and at what cost it can be achieved.

Hofstede, G. *Culture's Consequences: International Differences in Work-Related Values*. Thousand Oaks, Calif.: Sage, 1984. A foundation piece in the literature about culture, this research-based book discusses culturally based differences in values that affect the workplace. Aspects such as individualism, power, distance, masculinity, and uncertainty avoidance are examined.

Hubbard, E. E. *Measuring Diversity Results*. Petaluma, Calif.: Global Insights Publishing, 1997. This book provides practical guidance in measurement, a key aspect of diversity implementation.

Jamieson, D., and O'Mara, J. *Managing Workforce 2000: Gaining the Diversity Advantage*. San Francisco: Jossey-Bass, 1991. This pioneering book outlines a method for managing diversity using the authors flex management approach. A number of organizational examples demonstrating effective practices are provided.

Knowles, L., Prewitt, K. *Institutional Racism in America*. Englewood Cliffs, N.J.: Prentice Hall, 1969. This book gives a comprehensive account of the pervasiveness of racism in institutions in this society.

Loden, M., and Rosener, J. B. *Workforce America! Managing Employee Diversity as a Vital Resource*. Burr Ridge, Ill: Irwin, 1991. This foundation piece in the literature about diversity makes a case for creating an organization that capitalizes on the richness in differences. It offers an insightful look at the issues that emerge, as well as at managerial and organizational strategies to deal with them.

Pedersen, P. *A Handbook for Developing Multicultural Awareness*. Alexandria, Va.: American Association for Counseling and Development, 1988. This book written for counselors also serves as a resource for managers working with staff from other cultures as well as employees working with multicultural coworkers and customers.

Ponterotto, J. G., and Pedersen, P. B. *Preventing Prejudice: A Guide for Counselors and Educators*. Thousand Oaks, Calif.: Sage, 1993. This relevant and pragmatic book serves as an excellent resource for understanding the nature of prejudice and provides developmentally sequenced exercises for dealing with problems of prejudice.

Prasad, P., Mills, A. J., Elmes, M. B., and Prasad, A. (eds.). *Managing the Organizational Melting Pot: Dilemmas of Workplace Diversity*. Thousand Oaks, Calif.: Sage, 1997. This collection of writings provides an array of theoretical frameworks for illuminating the difficulties of workplace diversity.

Samovar, L. A., and Porter, R. E. *Intercultural Communication: A Reader.* Belmont, Calif.: Wadsworth, 1976. This anthology brings together a series of forty-four articles on culture in general as well as on specific cultures and aspects of intercultural communication. Both theoretical and practical information are included.

Thiederman, S. *Bridging Cultural Barriers for Corporate Success: How to Manage the Multicultural Work Force.* San Francisco: New Lexington Press, 1990. This handbook for cross-cultural communication gives practical information about motivating, attracting, interviewing, retaining, and training the multicultural workforce. This reader-friendly book is full of applicable examples, how-tos, and exercises for overcoming obstacles to intercultural communication.

Thomas, R. R. *Beyond Race and Gender: Unleashing the Power of Your Total Work Force by Managing Diversity.* New York: AMACOM, 1991. This book puts forth a fundamental plan for managing diversity, coupled with practical examples of how organizations capitalize on their diverse staffs. It includes a strategy for a cultural audit as well as an action plan for change.

Ting-Toomey, S., and Korzenny, F. (eds.). *Cross-Cultural Interpersonal Communication.* Thousand Oaks, Calif.: Sage, 1991. This collection of articles covers current research and theories in cross-cultural communication.

Turkewych, C., and Guerrerro-Klinoroski, H. *Intercultural Interviewing: The Key to Effective Hiring in a Multicultural Workforce.* Halle, Quebec: International Briefing Associates, 1992. By providing guidelines and critical incidents, this manual serves as a task-specific resource for managers, human resource personnel, and trainees regarding each stage of the interviewing process.

Books About African Americans

Chideya, F. *Don't Believe the Hype: Fighting Cultural Misinformation About African-Americans.* New York: Penguin Books, 1995. This book offers an array of factual information to refute many common misconceptions and stereotypes about African Americans. It is designed to give readers a chance to question the standard depictions of race in today's news media and popular press.

Davis, G., and Watson, G. *Black Life in Corporate America*. New York: Anchor Books, 1982. This book sheds light on the impact of American organizational culture on black employees.

Fernandez, J. *Racism and Sexism in Corporate Life*. San Francisco: New Lexington Books, 1981. This book discusses the findings of a major study of black and white men and women in the workplace, focusing on how racism and sexism affect their work life.

Gary, L. *Black Men*. Thousand Oaks, Calif.: Sage, 1981. This book discusses issues confronting black men in America today.

Grier, W. H., and Cobbs, P. M. *Black Rage*. New York: HarperCollins, 1991. This classic in the diversity field offers the views of two black psychiatrists on the inner conflicts and desperation of black life in the United States.

Hacker, A. *Two Nations: Black and White, Separate, Hostile, Unequal*. New York: Scribner, 1992. A fresh and human analysis of race relations in America is given in this book, which diagnoses the problems but offers no prescription for solutions.

Rodgers-Rose, L. *Black Women*. Thousand Oaks, Calif.: Sage, 1983. Issues and conditions confronting black women are discussed in this book.

Taylor, R. J., Jackson, J. S., and Chotters, L. M. (eds.). *Family Life in Black America*. Thousand Oaks, Calif.: Sage, 1997. This series of articles moves away from a deficit perspective and problem focus and offers information based on empirical data regarding diversity among today's African American families.

West, C. *Race Matters*. Boston: Beacon Press, 1993. In this book the author discusses the dynamics and impact of racism in America.

Williams, G. H. *Life on the Color Line*. New York: NAL/Dutton, 1995. This true story of a white boy who discovered he was black poignantly illustrates the effects of prejudice and discrimination in American life.

Work, J. W. *Race, Economics and Corporate America*. Wilmington, Del.: Scholarly Resources, 1984. This book explores the impact of socioeconomic factors and racism on the status of African Americans.

Books About Men and Women and Gender Differences

Astrachan, A. *How Men Feel*. New York: Anchor Books, 1988. How men feel about women is the topic of this book, which contains a number of chapters focusing on work relationships.

Farrell, W. *Why Men Are the Way They Are*. New York: McGraw-Hill, 1986. This book offers insights and understanding, not only about male behavior but also about male-female relationships.

Gilligan, C. *In a Different Voice: Psychological Theory and Women's Development*. Cambridge, Mass.: Harvard University Press, 1962. This book presents a seminal discussion of gender differences in moral and ethical development and the implications for the workplace.

Gray, J. *Men Are from Mars, Women Are from Venus: A Practical Guide for Improving Communication and Getting What You Want in Your Relationships*. New York: HarperCollins, 1992. This look at male-female differences argues that communication problems between the sexes are rooted in gender-related value differences.

Gutek, B. A. *Sex and the Work Place*. San Francisco: Jossey-Bass, 1985. This book examines a critical aspect of male-female interaction on the job—the impact of sexual behavior and harassment on women, men, and organizations. The issue is looked at from managerial, legal, psychological, and social perspectives.

Heim, P., and Galant, S. *Hardball for Women: Winning at the Game of Business*. Los Angeles: Lowell House, 1992. Differences between male and female leadership skills are the subject of this book. Tracing gender differences to the play of boys and girls, the authors apply these preferences to adult behaviors in the workplace.

Landrine, H., and Klonoff, E. A. *Discrimination Against Women: Prevalence, Consequences and Remedies*. Thousand Oaks, Calif.: Sage, 1997. The authors offer an empirically validated scale for measuring the health effects of sexism, and report their findings on the mental and physical health impacts of discrimination.

Lipman-Blumen, J. *Gender Roles and Power*. Englewood Cliffs, N.J.: Prentice Hall, 1984. This book explains the way in which the gender system is a foundation for all other power relationships.

Loden, M. *Feminine Leadership, or How to Succeed in Business Without Being One of the Boys*. New York: Times Books, 1985. This book delineates differences between male and female leadership styles and makes suggestions for enhancing the workplace.

Milwid, B. *Working with Men: Professional Women Talk About Power, Sexuality, and Ethics*. Hillsboro, Oreg.: Beyond Words, 1990. Interviews with 125 professional women provide a look at what it is like for women in the workplace. This book gives an insider's look at the pressures, problems, and hopes of women in the work world.

Morrison, A. M., White, R. P., and van Velson, E. *Breaking the Glass Ceiling*. Reading, Mass.: Addison-Wesley, 1987. Based on a study of executives, this book examines the factors that determine the success and failure of women in corporate America.

Pearson, J. C. *Gender and Communication*. Dubuque, Iowa: W. C. Brown, 1985. This book focuses on the gender gap in interactions, discussing the difficulties and differences in communication between men and women.

Powell, G. *Women and Men in Management: The Dynamics of Interaction*. Thousand Oaks, Calif.: Sage, 1988. In this book, the author downplays the importance of male-female differences.

Rosener, J. B. *America's Competitive Secret: Utilizing Women as a Management Strategy*. New York: Oxford University Press, 1995. This book describes the unique contribution of female professionals and explains why men and women are perceived and evaluated differently at work. It helps both men and women to understand the economic, social, and psychological impact of women and men as peers and competitors. It includes chapters on sexual static and how men and women feel.

Sargent, A. G. *Beyond Sex Roles*. St. Paul, Minn.: West, 1977. Through exercises and narrative explanations, the author and other contributors teach, raise awareness, and prod self-exploration about sex roles and about change in these roles.

Simons, G. F., and Weissman, G. D. *Men and Women: Partners at Work*. Los Altos, Calif.: Crisp Publications, 1990. The objective of this book is to help men and women approach each other openly, creatively, and with effective communication tools. Exercises and worksheets help readers identify and resolve gender issues that inhibit productivity and understanding.

Tannen, D. *You Just Don't Understand: Women and Men in Conversation*. New York: Morrow, 1991. In a down-to-earth, reader-friendly style, the author explains gender differences in communication that produce obstacles. Recognizing and understanding these differences can be a help in avoiding barriers to clear communication between men and women.

Tingley, J. *Genderflex: Men and Women Speaking Each Others' Language at Work*. New York: AMACOM, 1994. This book gives suggestions about overcoming the gender gap in work communication.

Books About Latinos

Condon, J. C. *Good Neighbors: Communication with the Mexicans*. Yarmouth, Mass.: Intercultural Press, 1985. In this concise book, the author describes how the cultures of the United States and Mexico differ, how Mexicans and North Americans misunderstand each other, and what can be done to bridge the gap. Vital information for those working with Mexicans is provided in a readable, interesting way.

Knouse, S. B., Rosenfeld, P., and Culbertson, A. (eds.). *Hispanics in the Workplace*. Thousand Oaks, Calif.: Sage, 1992. A comprehensive exploration of Hispanic employment factors, problems at work, support systems, and Hispanic women and work. Contributors deal with specific topics such as recruiting, training, and language barriers.

Kras, E. S. *Management in Two Cultures: Bridging the Gap Between U.S. and Mexican Managers.* Yarmouth, Maine: Intercultural Press, 1989. This book pinpoints the principal differences between Mexican and U.S. cultures and management styles that cause misunderstandings and conflict. It gives concrete recommendations to both U.S. and Mexican managers for dealing more effectively with each other.

Miranda, A. *The Chicano Experience: An Alternative Perspective.* Notre Dame, Ind.: University of Notre Dame Press, 1985. The social and economic conditions facing Mexican Americans are explained in this book.

Sharris, E. *Latinos: A Biography of the People.* New York: Norton, 1992. This book offers a deeper understanding of many Spanish-speaking cultures. The origin of the main groups, their history, and their current situations are told mainly through biographies of individuals and families.

Books About Other Groups

Althen, G. *American Ways: A Guide for Foreigners in the United States.* Yarmouth, Maine: Intercultural Press, 1988. This book is designed for those who want to understand the behaviors and values of Americans. In easy-to-understand language and clear examples, the author describes the basic characteristics of U.S. culture and offers suggestions for effective interactions with Americans.

Andres, T. *Understanding Filipino Values: A Management Approach.* Quezon City, Philippines: New Day, 1981. This book is a resource for understanding Filipino culture and values, with an emphasis on management issues.

Barker, R. G. *Adjustment to Physical Handicap and Illness: A Survey of the Social Psychology of Physique and Disability.* New York: Social Science Research Council, 1953. This book combines a theoretical and practical discussion of the social psychology of differently abled people. It also contains a chapter on employment.

Baylan, E. *Women and Disability*. Atlantic Highlands, N.J.: Zed Books, 1991. This book discusses the issues faced by women with disabilities.

Blumfeld, W. J., and Raymond, D. *Looking at Gay and Lesbian Life*. Boston: Beacon Press, 1988. Lesbian and gay lifestyles in the United States are examined and discussed in this book.

Condon, J. C. *With Respect to the Japanese: A Guide for Americans*. Yarmouth, Maine: Intercultural Press, 1984. In this handbook, the author discusses aspects of Japanese values and behavior that affect communications, business relations, and management styles. He goes on to make recommendations on how to deal with the Japanese during face-to-face encounters.

Fieg, J. P., and Mortlock, E. *A Common Core: Thais and Americans*. Yarmouth, Maine: Intercultural Press, 1989. Both commonalties and differences between Thai and American cultures are explained in this book. The authors go on to discuss the implications of the differences for people engaged in cross-cultural encounters on and off the job.

Fisher, G. *International Negotiations: A Cross-Cultural Perspective*. Yarmouth, Maine: Intercultural Press, 1980. By comparing how Japanese, Mexicans, French, and Americans reach agreements, the author demonstrates how culture influences the negotiation process and suggests a useful line of questioning and analysis for intercultural negotiation.

Gochenour, T. *Considering Filipinos*. Yarmouth, Maine: Intercultural Press, 1990. This intercultural handbook contrasts the values and perspectives of Filipinos and Americans and offers guidelines for successful interaction between these two groups. It gives suggestions for bridging cultural differences in social and workplace settings, as well as case studies showing cross-cultural dynamics in action.

Kitano, H. L., and Daniels, R. *Asian Americans: Emerging Minorities*. Englewood Cliffs, N.J.: Prentice Hall, 1988. This book focuses on the various Asian ethnic groups, discussing their experiences in America.

Lanier, A. R. *Living in the USA*. Yarmouth, Maine: Intercultural Press, 1988. This book is designed to help foreigners and newcomers understand the United States. It provides a guide to customs, courtesies, and caveats, and gives practical advice to anyone coming to the United States to live.

McLuhan, T. C. *Touch the Earth*. New York: Simon & Schuster, 1971. This book recollects the Native American way of life and contrasts it with mainstream American society and values.

Mead, M. *Culture and Commitment: A Study of the Generation Gap*. New York: Doubleday, 1970. This anthropologist's look at the generation gap explains the differences in views and perspectives between the young and the old.

Nelson, R. *Creating Acceptance for Handicapped People*. Springfield, Ill.: Thomas, 1978. This handbook is designed to teach the community to be supportive and accepting of people with disabilities, either physical or mental.

Nydell, M. K. *Understanding Arabs: A Guide for Westerners*. Yarmouth, Maine: Intercultural Press, 1987. This readable cross-cultural handbook gives a concise and insightful look at Arab culture. It dispels common Western misconceptions regarding Arab behavior and explains the values, beliefs, and practices of Arabs, particularly in terms of their impact on interactions with Europeans and North Americans.

Richmond, Y. *From Da to Yes: Understanding the East Europeans*. Yarmouth, Maine: Intercultural Press, 1995. Another in the InterActs series, this book offers help in understanding and dealing with people from Eastern Europe. It contains chapters on Poles, Czechs, Slovaks, Hungarians, Romanians, Moldovans, Bulgarians, Serbs, Croats, Slovenes, Albanians, Ukrainians, and others.

Richmond, Y. *From Nyet to Da: Understanding the Russians*. Yarmouth, Maine: Intercultural Press, 1992. This succinctly written book is a cross-cultural guide for dealing with Russians. The author outlines ways of responding most effectively to Russians on a personal level as well as in business.

Root, M.P.P. *Filipino Americans: Transforming Identity*. Thousand Oaks, Calif.: Sage, 1997. This collection of articles from historians, social workers, psychologists, educators, and ethnic scholars addresses issues such as ethnic identity, relationships, and mental health.

Sagarin, E. (ed.). *The Other Minorities*. Waltham, Mass.: Xerox College, 1971. Non-ethnic minorities, such as the differently abled, are the subjects in this collection of articles.

Shahar, L., and Kurz, D. *Border Crossings: American Interactions with Israelis*. Yarmouth, Maine: Intercultural Press, 1995. In case studies based on real situations, the authors show Americans and Israelis attempting to communicate across cultural barriers. They also offer coping strategies and exercises that help readers to choose those that are most appropriate for their own personal style.

Stewart, E. C. *American Cultural Patterns: A Cross-Cultural Perspective*. Yarmouth, Maine: Intercultural Press, 1972. Using the value orientation framework of Kluckholn and Strodtbeck, the author examines American patterns of thinking and behaving. He goes on to analyze the assumptions about human nature and the physical world that underlie these values, and to compare and contrast them with those of other cultures.

Wenzhong, H., and Grove, C. L. *Encountering the Chinese: A Guide for Americans*. Yarmouth, Maine: Intercultural Press, 1991. This useful book goes beyond description to explain Chinese behavior. It provides a cross-cultural analysis that can guide Westerners toward more effective relationships with the Chinese.

Winfeld, L., and Spielman, S. *Straight Talk About Gays in the Workplace: Creating an Inclusive Environment for Everyone in Your Organization*. New York: American Management Association, 1995. This candid book brings the myths and facts about gays out into the open and offers a clear look at how companies can include issues of sexual orientation in their nondiscrimination and diversity management programs.

Books About Customer Service and Marketing in a Diverse Environment

Ricks, D. A. *Blunders in International Business*. Cambridge, Mass.: Blackwell Publishers, 1993. This book, based on the premise that mistakes often teach more than successes, focuses on examples of blunders that illustrate the cost of not understanding cultural differences in business. It is rich with anecdotes and stories that demonstrate the point.

Rossman, M. L. *Multicultural Marketing: Selling to a Diverse America*. New York: AMACOM, 1994. In this book the author describes the $500 billion market represented by America's so-called minorities, the most important consumer growth area in the United States. She then goes on to explain differences among the segments of this market and how to reach them.

Shames, G. W., and Glover, W. G. *World Class Service*. Yarmouth, Maine: Intercultural Press, 1989. This book explores the implications of world-class service from four major operational perspectives—business strategy, marketing, human resource development, and customer contact, using specific organizations and cases. It emphasizes cross-cultural management as a key priority in the operational phases of international or domestic cross-cultural business operations.

Thiederman, S. *Profiting in America's Multicultural Marketplace: How to Do Business Across Cultural Lines*. San Francisco: New Lexington Books, 1991. In practical, readable terms, the author explains cultural effects on person-to-person behavior and how to communicate effectively with people of different backgrounds. The author also gives anecdotes and tests that involve and teach.

Structured Experiences, Games, and Training Activities

Bafa Bafa: Cross-Cultural Orientation. Gary R. Shirts, P.O. Box 910, Del Mar, Calif. 92014, (619)755-0272. This experiential activity simulates the contact between two very different cultures, Alpha and Beta. The activity is structured so that participants learn through direct simulated experience and then apply that learning to real-life situations. (*Rafa Rafa*, a simplified version for children in grades 5 through 8, is also available.)

Barnga: A Simulation Game on Cultural Clashes. Sivasailam Thiagarajan, Intercultural Press, P.O. Box 700, Yarmouth, Maine 04096, (207) 846-5168. Through playing a simple card game in small groups, participants experience the effect of simulated cultural differences on human interaction. This activity is easy to run in a relatively short time.

The Diversity Game. Quality Educational Development, 41 Central Park West, New York, N.Y. 10023, (212)724-3335. This multiplayer board game provides insights, raises awareness, and stimulates discussion about diversity issues in the workplace. Questions focus on real workplace issues such as communication, motivation, reward, recognition, respect, and trust in the context of gender, race, and cultural diversity.

The Diversity Tool Kit. Lee Gardenswartz and Anita Rowe. Irwin Professional Publishing, 1333 Burr Ridge Parkway, Burr Ridge, Ill. 60521, (800) 634-3966. This resource provides over 100 training activities in reproducible, ready-to-use format on aspects such as stereotypes and prejudices, culture, team building, and hiring and recruitment.

Diversophy. Multus, Inc., 46 Treetop Lane, Suite 200, San Mateo, Calif. 94402-3234, (415)342-2040. This board game is designed to be played by line managers, supervisors, administrative personnel, salespeople, customer service representatives, and senior executives. Easy to play, the game delivers thought-provoking information, deals with critical attitudes, and teaches useful skills for meeting the challenges of diversity.

Ecotonos. Dianne Hofner-Saphiere and Nipporica Associates. Intercultural Press, P.O. Box 700, Yarmouth, Maine, (207)846-5168. This simulation deals with problem solving and decision making in multicultural groups.

The Global Diversity Game. Quality Educational Development, 41 Central Park West, New York, N.Y. 10023, (212)724-3335. In this board game, teams answer questions on demographics, jobs, legislation, and society as they relate to the global business environment. Cross-cultural and transnational information is highlighted, stimulating a dynamic exchange of knowledge and experience between participants.

Healthcare Diversity. Suzanne Salimbene and George Simons, Maltus Inc. and George Simons International, 46 Treetop Lane, Suite 200, San Mateo, Cailf. 94402, (415)342-2040. This interactive board game helps participants learn about diversity in health care.

Redundancia. Dianne Hofner-Saphiere and Nipporica Associates. 10072 Buena Vista Drive, Conifer, Colo. 80433, (303)838-1798. This short, effective simulation helps people understand the challenges faced by people attempting to communicate in a second language.

Diversity Videos and Films

Bill Cosby on Prejudice. Budget Films, 4590 Santa Monica Blvd., Los Angeles, Calif. 90029, (213)660-0187. This film presents a monologue on prejudice by Bill Cosby.

Bridges: Skills for Managing a Diverse Workforce. BNA Communications, 9439 Key West Ave., Rockville, Md. 20850, (800)253-6067. This eight-module video-based program is designed to train managers and supervisors in managing diverse workers. It raises awareness about cultural, racial, and gender differences and presents the skills to deal with them. The series includes manuals for trainees and participants.

Bridging Cultural Barriers: Managing Ethnic Diversity in the Workplace. Barr Films, 12801 Schabarum Ave., P.O. Box 7878, Irwindale, Calif. 91706-7878, (800)234-7878. This half-hour film featuring Sondra Thiederman teaches about the effective management of diverse workers through simulated examples of a manager resolving situations with two culturally different staff members. Vignettes are interspersed with brief lectures by Thiederman.

The Cost of Intolerance. BNA Communications, 9439 Key West Ave., Rockville, Md. 20850-3396, (800)233-6067. This six-unit video program helps employees to improve customer service and increase sales by valuing diverse customers. Issues such as handling customers who speak with thick accents and overcoming subtle biases and stereotypes are dealt with through realistic vignettes.

Cultural Diversity in the Hospital Setting: Fostering Understanding and Developing Cross-Cultural Management Skills. Sondra Thiederman, 1993. Distributed by Hospital Educational Services, P.O. Box 396, La Jolla, Calif. 92038, (800)858-4478. This two-hour video of an actual workshop with employees of Green Hospital, Scripps Clinic, La Jolla, California, focuses on intercultural communication. Many examples and practical suggestions are given.

Dealing with Diversity. American Media Incorporated, 4900 University Ave., West Des Moines, Iowa 50266-6769, (800)262-2557. This video training program helps employees to deal with diversity by understanding how others want to be treated. It focuses on understanding and respecting individual differences, and improving communication by asking questions and listening.

Diverse Teams at Work. corVision, 1339 Barclay Blvd., Buffalo Grove, Ill. 60089, (800)537-3130. This video, based on the book of the same title, demonstrates the impact of the many dimensions of diversity on the interactions of a work team. Understanding of these differences is developed as a critical step toward building respect between people of different backgrounds.

Faces. Salinger Films, 1635 12th St., Santa Monica, Calif. 90404, (310)450-1300. This one-minute, unnarrated video shows a kaleidoscope of human faces of different sexes, races, and ages merging and complementing each other to form an integrative whole. By showing the individual worth of each face as well as its contribution to the total picture, the video demonstrates that we are all unique, yet we share a common bond.

Getting Along: Words of Encouragement. Cross Cultural Communications, 4585 48th St., San Diego, Calif. 92114, (800)858-4478. In four and a half minutes of printed messages and music, this video reminds people to work and live together with open hearts and open minds.

Let's Talk Diversity. American Media Incorporated, 4900 University Ave., West Des Moines, Iowa 50266-6769, (800)262-2557. This video training program helps all employees to understand how values, attitudes, and behaviors affect others. It also helps them recognize biases and stereotypes based on gender, race, religion, age, culture, disability, and lifestyle.

Living and Working in America. Via Press, 400 E. Evergreen Blvd., Suite 314, Vancouver, Wash. 98660, (800)944-8421. A comprehensive three-volume audiovisual series for training nonnative speakers of English in communication skills needed for supervisory and management positions in the multicultural workforce. Includes video scenes, textbook, audio-tapes, and an instructor's manual with experiential learning activities.

Managing Diversity. CRM Films, 2233 Faraday Ave., Carlsbad, Calif. 92008, (800)421-0833. This film combines dramatizations of information from experts in the field to focus on diversity issues such as stereotyping and communication as well as on differences in perception regarding teamwork, power, and authority. It ends with a useful list of things people can do to improve communication in a diverse environment. A guide is included.

Managing a Multicultural Workforce: The Mosaic Workplace. Films for the Humanities and Sciences, P.O. Box 2053, Princeton, N.J. 08543-2053, (800)257-5126. This training program of ten videos addresses the issues of the diverse workplace. It covers topics such as understanding different cultural values and styles, men and women working together, and success strategies for minorities.

The Multicultural Customer. Salinger Films, 1635 12th St., Santa Monica, Calif. 90404, (310)450-1300. This video helps customer service staff to understand the dynamics of cross-cultural communication and get beyond barriers to establishing positive relationships with diverse customers. It shows vignettes of typical customer-staff interactions and gives tips for providing top-notch service to a diverse population.

Sandcastle: A Film About Teamwork and Diversity. Salinger Films, 1635 12th St., Santa Monica, Calif. 90404, (310)450-1300. Teamwork and the contribution of each diverse team member is illustrated in this Academy Award–winning, unnarrated thirteen-minute video. A unique story about the building of a sandcastle, the film demonstrates the value of diversity.

Serving Customers with Disabilities. Salinger Films, 1635 12th St., Santa Monica, Calif. 90404, (310)450-1300. This film offers etiquette and cus-tomer service skills to help employees serve customers with disabilities more effectively.

A Tale of "O." Goodmeasure, Inc., P.O. Box 3004, Cambridge, Mass. 02139. This film and video deals with differentness by showing how a few O's learn to function in organizations made up of X's.

True Colors. Coronet/MTI Film and Video, 420 Academy Drive, Northbrook, Ill. 60062, (800)777-2400. In this provocative edition of ABC's *Prime Time*, host Diane Sawyer follows two college-educated men in their mid-thirties, one black, one white, as they involve themselves in a variety of everyday situations to test levels of prejudice based on skin color. The results are startling and unsettling.

Valuing Diversity. Copeland Griggs Productions, 302 23rd Ave., San Francisco, Calif. 94121, (415)668-4200. This seven-part film and video series for managers and other employees focuses on the advantages inherent in diversity. Segments deal with issues such as managing and supervising differences, upward mobility in a multicultural organization, and communicating across cultures. The series includes users' guides.

West Meets East in Japan. Pyramid Film and Video, Box 1048, Santa Monica, Calif. 90406, (800)421-2304. This culture-specific video lets you experience Japanese culture from the point of view of an outsider learning the norms of Japanese etiquette. A study guide is included.

Why Do We Kick a Brother or a Sister When They're Down? The Riverbend Press, P.O. Box 586, Concord, Mass. 01742, (508)371-2664. This powerful videotape is the true story of childhood friends and the destructive influences of classism and other prejudices. This training tool about human relations is especially useful in dealing with valuing differences.

A Winning Balance. BNA Communications, 9439 Key West Ave., Rockville, Md. 20850, (800)233-6067. This video-based training program introduces the topic of diversity and its importance to all employees. It goes on to deal with attitudes toward difference, the impact of biases, becoming a diversity change agent, and making a personal commitment. Trainer and participant manuals are included.

Working Together: Managing Cultural Diversity. Crisp Publications, 1200 Hamilton Ct., Menlo Park, Calif. 94025, (800)442-7477. This video-book program teaches how to work productively in a multicultural environment. Users learn how to manage their attitudes and communication in interactions with people from other cultures. The kit includes a leader's guide.

Diversity Assessment Tools and Instruments

Grote, K. *Diversity Awareness Profile* and *Diversity Awareness Profile, Manager's Version*. Pfeiffer, 350 Sansome Street, San Francisco, Calif. 94104, (415) 433-1740. A forty-item questionnaire places respondents in one of five categories on the Diversity Awareness Spectrum. The profile suggests action steps and includes notes for trainers.

Halverson, C. B. *Cultural Context Work Style Inventory*. School for International Training, Experiment in International Living, Brattleboro, Vt., (802)254-6098. This self-scored, twenty-item questionnaire is designed for self-understanding based on the high-low context framework of Edward Hall. It includes background information, charts, and a bibliography.

Kelley, C., and Meyers, J. *The Cross-Cultural Adaptability Inventory*. C. Kelley and J. Meyers, 2500 Torey Pines Rd., La Jolla, Calif. 92037, (619)453-8165. This self-scoring instrument is for people planning to work and live abroad. It measures four critical dimensions of cross-cultural adaptability. A manual is included.

Overseas Assignment Inventory (OAI). Moran, Stahl & Boyer, International Division, 900 28th St., Boulder, Colo. 80303, (303)449-8440. This self-response questionnaire measures fifteen attitudes and attributes important to cross-cultural adjustment. Resulting in a profile of cross-cultural adaptability, this standardized and normed instrument can be applied in selection, placement, counseling, workforce planning, career development, and self-selection.

The Questions of Diversity: Assessment Tools for Organizations and Individuals (1990). George Simons, ODT Incorporated, P.O. Box 134, Amherst, Mass. 01004, (413)549-1293. This tool contains nine surveys that assess personal and organizational issues of diversity in the workplace. These instruments are intended as learning tools.

Periodicals, Journals, and Newsletters

Cross-Cultural Research: The Journal of Comparative Social Science. Sage Publications, Inc., P.O. Box 5084, Thousand Oaks, Calif. 91359,

(805)499-9774. This scholarly journal publishes refereed studies pertaining to cross-cultural issues in the social and behavioral sciences.

Cultural Diversity at Work. The GilDeane Group, 13751 Lake City Way NE, Suite 106, Seattle, Wash. 98125-8612, (206)362-0336. This bimonthly newsletter offers articles and resource reviews on relevant and topical issues facing today's diverse organizations. Its practical focus aims at preparing the reader for "managing, training and conducting business in the global age." Subscription also includes eleven monthly issues of *The Diversity Networker,* which lists upcoming diversity conferences, seminars, and events.

Culturally Competent Care. Inter-Face International, 3821 East State St., Suite 197, Rockford, Ill. 61108, (815) 965-7535. This bimonthly newsletter provides concrete, culture-specific information to help providers reach out to patients from other cultures. While intended for those in health care, its information can also be of value to customer service staff and managers in other cultural settings.

The COSSMHO Reporter. The National Coalition of Hispanic Health and Human Service Organizations, 1501 Sixteenth St. NW, Washington, D.C. 20036, (202)389-5000. This biannual newsletter provides information about issues of health care for Hispanics.

The Diversity Marketing Outlook. The GilDeane Group, 13751 Lake City Way NE, Suite 106, Seattle, Wash. 98125-8612, (206)362-0336. This quarterly magazine focuses on advertising and marketing to today's increasingly diverse consumer base. It features examples of creative approaches and new developments in the arena of multicultural marketing.

Journal of Cross-Cultural Psychology. Sage Publications, Inc., P.O. Box 5084, Thousand Oaks, Calif. 91359, (805)499-9774. This journal presents behavioral and social research focusing on psychological phenomena as differentially influenced by culture.

Managing Diversity. Jamestown Area Labor Management Committee, Inc., P.O. Box 819, Jamestown, N.Y. 14702-0819, (716)665-3654. This monthly newsletter directed at business leaders and managers offers a series of articles on pertinent issues faced in leading and managing diversity organizations. Through thoughtful articles and practical approaches it challenges and educates the reader.

Web Sites and Other Resources

Cultural Diversity Hotwire [http://www.diversityhotwire.com]. This Web site of *Cultural Diversity at Work* newsletter provides an article of the month, abstracts of newsletter articles, and a catalogue of books, videos, and back issues, as well as a networking/learning events calendar.

Inter-Face International [http://www.cmihub.com/†/InterFaceInt.htm]. This Web site offers a listing of diversity products and services for the health care field.

Multicultural Calendar. Creative Cultural Communications, 12300 Contra Costa Blvd., Suite 270, Pleasant Hill, Calif. 94523, (800)883-4072. This wall calendar containing twelve original ethnic artworks lists holidays and cultural events of a wide variety of religions and cultures.

Multicultural Resource Calendar. Amherst Educational Publishing, 30 Blue Hills Rd., Amherst, Mass. 01002, (800)865-5549. This award winning calendar educates staff by increasing awareness about the contributions of people of over 35 different backgrounds, and holidays of over 35 groups.

National Multicultural Institute [http://www.nmci.org/nmci/links.htm]. This site provides many multicultural Web links.

The 1998 Health Practitioner's Multi-Cultural Resource Calendar. Suzanne Salimbene, Amherst Educational Publishing, 30 Blue Hills Road, Amherst, Mass. 01002, (800)865-5548. This calendar presents monthly health care tips and provides a separate resource section on health care characteristics of Hispanic, Asian, African American, and Native American patients.

Notes

Introduction

1. Suzanne Salimbene and Jack W. Graczykowski, *When Two Cultures Meet: American Medicine and the Cultures of Diverse Patient Populations*. Hawthorne, Calif.: Inter-Face International, 1995, p. 1.

2. "Minorities Are Majority in 2000 Areas," *The Los Angeles Times*, June 9, 1993.

3. California Department of Health Services, "Culturally Appropriate and Linguistically Competent Services." In *Expanding Medi-Cal Managed Care*. Sacramento: California Department of Health Services, 1994, p. 45.

4. Nathaniel Hawthorne, *The Custom House*. Mattituck, N.Y.: Amereon, 1976.

5. Salimbene and Graczykowski, *When Two Cultures Meet*, pp. 5–6.

6. Terence Monmaney, "Ethnicities' Medical Views Vary, Study Says," *The Los Angeles Times*, Sept. 13, 1995, pp. B1, B3.

7. Suzanne Salimbene and Jack W. Graczykowski, *Culture, Traditional Medicine and Your Chinese/American Patient*. Hawthorne, Calif.: Inter-Face International, 1995, p. 21.

8. Kim Witte and Kelly Morrison, "Intercultural and Cross-Cultural Health Communication." In R. L. Weisman (ed.), *Intercultural Communication Theory*. Thousand Oaks, Calif.: Sage, 1995, p. 220.

Chapter One

1. "Latinos, Asians to Lead Rise in U.S. Population," *The Los Angeles Times*, Mar. 14, 1996.

2. "The New Face of America," *Time*, Fall 1993 (Special Issue), pp. 14–15.

3. "The New Face of America," pp. 14–15.

4. Marlene Rossman, *Multicultural Marketing: Selling to a Diverse America*. New York: AMACOM, 1994, p. 3.

5. Rossman, *Multicultural Marketing*, p. 3.

6. "Minorities Are Majority in 2,000 Areas."

7. "Serving Diverse Customers," *The Los Angeles Times*, Oct. 23, 1994.

8. "Serving Diverse Customers."

9. Suzanne Salimbene, "Cultural Competency and the Expansion and Transition of Medi-Cal to Managed Care Program." Unpublished material, Inter-Face International, 1995.

10. "Serving Diverse Customers."

Chapter Two

1. Maya Angelou, *Wouldn't Take Nothing for My Journey Now*. New York: Random House, 1993, pp. 124–125.

2. Tabiri Chukunta, personal communication, 1994.

3. Marilyn Loden and Judy B. Rosener, *Workforce America!* Burr Ridge, Ill.: Irwin, 1991, pp. 18–19.

4. Deborah Tannen, *You Just Don't Understand*. New York: Ballantine Books, 1990.

5. Aguirre-Molina and Molina, "Ethnic/Racial Populations and Worksite Health Promotion," p. 796.

6. Richard Brislin, *Understanding Culture's Influence on Behavior*. Orlando: Harcourt Brace, 1993, pp. 326, 347.

7. Marlene Rossman, *Multicultural Marketing*, p. 160.

8. Janet Elsea, *The Four-Minute Sell*. New York: Simon & Schuster, 1984.

9. Alicia H. Minnel, Lynn E. Browne, James McEneaney, and Geoffrey M. B. Tootell, "Mortgage Lending in Boston: Interpreting HMDA Data," Federal Reserve Bank of Boston, unpublished.

10. Jill Klessig, "The Effect of Values and Culture on Life Support Decisions," *The Western Journal of Medicine*, 1992, *157*(3).

11. Aguirre-Molina and Molina, "Ethnic/Racial Populations and Worksite Health Promotion," p. 794.

12. Aguirre-Molina and Molina, "Ethnic/Racial Populations and Worksite Health Promotion," p. 794.

13. Nikki Katalanos, "When Yes Means No: Verbal and Non-Verbal Communication of Southeast Asian Refugees in the New Mexico Health Care System," unpublished master's thesis, University of New Mexico, May 1994.

14. Aguirre-Molina and Molina, "Ethnic/Racial Populations and Worksite Health Promotion," p. 792.

15. Kaiser Permanente, *A Provider's Handbook on Culturally Competent Care: Latino Population*. Oakland, Calif.: Kaiser Permanente National Diversity Council, 1996, p. 12.

16. Douglas Clement, "Border Crossings: Refugees Travel Difficult Route to Health Care," *Minnesota Medicine*, 1992, *75*, p. 26.

17. Aguirre-Molina and Molina, "Ethnic/Racial Populations and Worksite Health Promotion," p. 792.

Chapter Three

1. John E. Jones, personal communication, 1977.

2. Philip R. Harris and Robert T. Moran, *Managing Cultural Differences*, 2nd ed. Houston: Gulf, 1987, pp.190–195.

3. Edward Hall, *The Hidden Dimension*. New York: Doubleday, 1966, pp. 159–160.

4. Salimbene and Graczykowski, *Culture, Traditional Medicine and Your Chinese/American Patient*, p. 15.

5. Siok-Hian Tay Kelley, "Hospitals' Staffs Adapt to Patients' Cultural Differences," *The Los Angeles Times*, July 25, 1990.

6. Kelley, "Hospitals' Staffs Adapt to Patients' Cultural Differences."

7. Jaime Wurzel, *Toward Multiculturalism: A Reader in Multicultural Education*. Yarmouth, Maine: Intercultural Press, 1988.

8. J. B. Rotter, "Generalized Expectations for Internal and External Control of Reinforcement," *Psychological Monograph*, 1966, 80.

Chapter Four

1. Pellegrino, Edmund. "Ethnicity and Healing." In *Trials, Tribulations, and Celebrations: African-American Perspectives on Health, Illness, Aging, and Loss*, edited by Marian Gray Secundy with Lois LaCivita Nixon, xix. Reprinted with permission of Intercultural Press, Inc., Yarmouth, Maine. Copyright 1992. Pellegrino is director of the Center for the Advanced Study of Ethics at Georgetown University.

2. Dwayne C. Turner, "The Role of Culture in Chronic Illness," *American Behavioral Scientist*, 1996, 39(6), 717.

3. Arthur Kleinman, Leon Eisenberg, and Byron Good, "Culture, Illness and Care," *Annals of Internal Medicine*, 88(2), p. 252.

4. Salimbene and Graczykowski, *Culture, Traditional Medicine and Your Chinese/American Patient*, pp. 17.

5. Kaiser Permanente National Diversity Council, *A Provider's Handbook on Culturally Competent Care*. Oakland, Calif.: Kaiser Permanente National Diversity Council, 1996.

6. Turner, "The Role of Culture in Chronic Illness," p. 717.

7. Turner, "The Role of Culture in Chronic Illness," p. 717.

8. Turner, "The Role of Culture in Chronic Illness," p. 717.

9. Mary Dee Hacker, personal communication, 1997.

10. "Health Care for New Americans: Blending Traditional and Western Medicine, Minnesota Medicine Interviews Patricia Walker, M.D.," *Minnesota Medicine*, 1992, 75, p. 11.

11. "HMO to Offer Acupuncture: It May Be First in State to Do So," *The Los Angeles Times*, Apr. 23, 1997, pp. D1, D11.

12. "Meditation and Healing," USA Today, July 31, 1997, p. 1.

13. Lillian S. Lew, "Understanding the Southeast Asian Health Care Consumer: Bridges and Barriers," In March of Dimes Birth Defects Foundation, Birth Defects: Original Article Series, 1990, 26(6), p. 152.

14. National Coalition of Hispanic Health and Human Service Organizations, Delivering Preventative Health Care to Hispanics: A Manual for Providers. Washington, D.C.: National Coalition of Hispanic Health and Human Service Organizations, 1990, p. 58.

15. Lew, "Understanding the Southeast Asian Health Care Consumer," p. 152.

16. "Health Care for New Americans," p. 11.

17. Dedra Buchwald, Sanjiv Panwala, and Thomas M. Hooton, "Use of Traditional Health Practices by Southeast Asian Refugees in a Primary Care Clinic," The Western Journal of Medicine, 1992, 156(5), p. 508.

18. Katalanos, "When Yes Means No."

19. Buchwald, Panwala, and Hooton, "Use of Traditional Health Practices by Southeast Asian Refugees in a Primary Care Clinic," p. 508.

20. Loudell F. Snow, "Traditional Health Beliefs and Practices Among Lower Class Black Americans," The Western Journal of Medicine, 1983, 139(6), p. 821.

21. Edith Stanley, "In with the New, but the Old Stays," The Los Angeles Times, June 19, 1997.

22. Edith Stanley, "In with the New, but the Old Stays."

23. B. Perrone, H. Stockel, and V. Kreuger (eds.), Medicine Women. Norman: University of Oklahoma Press, 1989, p. 29.

24. National Coalition of Hispanic Health and Human Service Organizations, Delivering Preventative Health Care to Hispanics, p. 58.

25. Katalanos, "When Yes Means No."

26. Snow, "Traditional Health Beliefs and Practices Among Lower Class Black Americans," pp. 820–828.

27. Katalanos, "When Yes Means No."

28. Verona C. Gordon, Irene M. Matousek, and Theresa A. Lang, "Southeast Asian Refugees: Life in America," *American Journal of Nursing*, Nov. 1980, pp. 2031–2036.

29. National Coalition of Hispanic Health and Human Service Organizations, *Delivering Preventative Health Care to Hispanics*, p. 50a.

30. Gordon, Matousek, and Lang, Nov. 1980, p. 2035.

31. Elaine Vandeventer, personal communication, 1997.

32. Barbara A. Koenig and Jan Gates-Williams, "Understanding Cultural Difference in Caring for Dying Patients," *The Western Journal of Medicine*, 1995, *163*(3), 244.

33. Koenig and Gates-Williams, "Understanding Cultural Difference in Caring for Dying Patients," p. 244.

34. Klessig, "The Effect of Values and Culture on Life Support Decisions," p. 366.

35. Klessig, "The Effect of Values and Culture on Life Support Decisions," p. 316.

36. Klessig, "The Effect of Values and Culture on Life Support Decisions," p. 316.

37. Klessig, "The Effect of Values and Culture on Life Support Decisions," p. 316.

38. Koenig and Gates-Williams, "Understanding Cultural Difference in Caring for Dying Patients," p. 244.

39. Klessig, "The Effect of Values and Culture on Life Support Decisions," p. 316.

40. Klessig, "The Effect of Values and Culture on Life Support Decisions," p. 316.

41. Deborah Harris-Abbot, "Variations in Cultural Attitudes Toward Autopsies," *Second Opinion*, 1994, *19*(4), 92.

42. Koenig and Gates-Williams, "Understanding Cultural Difference in Caring for Dying Patients," p. 244.

43. Gordon, Matousek, and Lang, "Southeast Asian Refugees," pp. 2031–2036.

44. Lew, "Understanding the Southeast Asian Health Care Consumer," pp. 147–154.

45. Klessig, "The Effect of Values and Culture on Life Support Decisions," p. 366.

46. Kim Witte and Kelly Morrison, "Intercultural and Cross-Cultural Health Communication: Understanding People and Motivating Healthy Behaviors," in Richard L. Wiseman (ed.), *Intercultural Communication Theory*. Thousand Oaks, Calif.: Sage, 1995, pp. 232–234.

47. Y. Beyene, "Medical Disclosure and Refugees: Telling Bad News to Ethiopian Patients," *Western Journal of Medicine*, 1992, p. 330.

48. M. Brod and S. Heurtin-Roberts, "Older Russian Émigrés and Medical Care," *Western Journal of Medicine*, 1992, p. 334.

Chapter Five

1. National Coalition of Hispanic Health and Human Services Organizations, *Delivering Preventative Health Care to Hispanics: A Manual for Providers*, p. 76.

2. Katalanos, "When Yes Means No," p. 33.

3. Katalanos, "When Yes Means No," p. 28.

4. Jorge Cherbosque, personal communication.

5. Merille Campbell Glover, "Food Service Manages Cultural Diversity," *California Hospitals*, July/Aug. 1991, p. 16.

6. *Speedy Spanish for Nursing Personnel*. Santa Barbara, Calif.: Baja Books, 1988; *Speedy Spanish for Medical Personnel*. Santa Barbara, Calif.: Baja Books, 1988; *Speedy Spanish for Physical Therapists*. Santa Barbara, Calif.: Baja Books, 1988. Baja Books can be reached at Box 4151, Santa Barbara, CA 93140.

7. Joseph Westermeyer, "Working with an Interpreter in Psychiatric Assessment and Treatment," *The Journal of Nervous and Mental Disease*, 1990, *178*(12), 748.

8. Adapted from Katalanos, "When Yes Means No," pp. 52–53. Reprinted with permission by Nikki Katalanos.

9. Lee Gardenswartz and Anita Rowe, *Managing Diversity: A Complete Desk Reference and Planning Guide*. Burr Ridge, Ill.: Irwin, 1993, 72–73.

10. Katalanos, "When Yes Means No," pp. 44–46.

11. Shotsy Faust and Robert Drichey, "Working with Interpreters," *The Journal of Family Practice*, 1986, 22(25), 136.

12. Elois Ann Berlin and William C. Fowkes Jr., "A Teaching Framework for Cross-Cultural Health Care," *The Western Journal of Medicine*, 1983, 139(6), 934.

13. Berlin and Fowkes, "A Teaching Framework for Cross-Cultural Health Care," pp. 934–935.

14. Toni Tripp-Reimer, Pamela J. Brink, and Judith M. Saunders, "Cultural Assessment: Content and Process," *Nursing Outlook*, 1984, 32(2), 81.

15. Douglas Clement, "Border Crossings: Refugees Travel Difficult Route to Health Care," *Minnesota Medicine*, 1992, 75, 28.

Chapter Six

1. Elaine Woo, "Can Racial Stereotypes Psych Out Students?" *The Los Angeles Times*, Dec. 11, 1995.

2. Farai Chedya, *Don't Believe the Hype*. New York: Penguin Books, 1995, pp. 155–156.

Chapter Seven

1. Stratford Sherman, "How Tomorrow's Best Leaders Are Learning Their Stuff," *Fortune*, Nov. 27, 1995, p. 92.

2. Information about Sisters of Providence Health System (SPHS) gathered from personal interviews with organization staff members.

3. Mark Meyer, personal communication, 1997.

4. Information on St. Francis Hospital gathered from personal interviews with organization staff members.

5. Sherman, "How Tomorrow's Best Leaders Are Learning Their Stuff," p. 92.

6. Sherman, "How Tomorrow's Best Leaders Are Learning Their Stuff," p. 92.

7. Information about Sisters of Providence Health System (SPHS) gathered from personal interviews with organization staff members.

8. Mary Kay Ash, personal communication, 1985.

9. Meyer, personal communication, 1997.

10. Patricia Digh, "Shades of Gray in the Global Marketplace," HRM Magazine, April 1997, pp. 91–98.

11. Digh, "Shades of Gray in the Global Marketplace," pp. 91–98.

12. Digh, "Shades of Gray in the Global Marketplace," pp. 91–98.

13. Digh, "Shades of Gray in the Global Marketplace," pp. 91–98.

14. Digh, "Shades of Gray in the Global Marketplace," pp. 91–98.

Index

W

Walker, P., 83
Washington state, 213–220
Watson, G., 228
Waxler-Morrison, N., 223
Web sites resource list, 244
Weissman, G. D., 231
Wenzhong, H., 235
West, C., 228
Western medicine: and folk or traditional medicine, 68, 78, 81, 85, 94, 213; and other cultures, 60–61, 81, 157; views of illness and health, 67–70, 132
White people (Anglos), 91–92; stereotypes about, 140, 147, 199
White, R. P., 230
Williams, G. H., 228
Winfeld, L., 235
Wiseman, R. L., 223
Witchcraft. *See* Folk or traditional medicine
Witte, K., 93
Women: abuse and assault survivors, 44; attitudes about touching, 106, 133–134; marketing health care services to, 11, 12, 89, 218–219; mentoring, 161–162, 206–210; resource books about, 228, 229–231, 233; speaking styles of, 18, 111, 213; status of, 72. *See also* Childbirth and prenatal care
Women health care providers, 217–218; patient preference for, 18, 19, 73; progress of, 200; using professional titles of, 109. *See also* Nurses; Physicians
Work experience: diversity and value of, 30, 58; seniority, 33–34, 158–159

Work habits and practices: cultural aspects of, 58–59, 61; and performance evaluation, 57, 168, 169, 170
Work, J. W., 229
Workforce populations: access to information, 77–78; accountability and flexibility of, 156–158, 168–169, 216; assessing customer services by, 181, 184, 185–186; cultural learning from your, 114, 116; demographics questionnaire, 3, 6; discrimination conditions within, 19, 194; ethnic makeup of, 199–200, 215, 227; ethnicity and health risks, 30; and external locus of control, 75–76; hiring community member, 153, 198–199; hourly and salaried, 31; interpreters and bicultural, 127–130, 131, 165–166, 168; management and nonmanagement, 32, 108, 238; organizational categories within, 15, 30–34; privacy values of, 74, 77; reward systems and incentives, 165, 168–169; scheduling, 31, 209, 217; status values in, 71–72, 78; teamwork in, 33, 76–77, 239; translators and bilingual, 130–132, 165, 183, 191–192, 204–205. *See also* Organizational dimensions of diversity; *specific ethnic groups*
World views. *See* Control, external or internal locus of; Ethnocentrism
Wu, E., 161–162

Y

Yakima Indians, 213–214
Yes-equals-no dilemma, 45, 104, 112, 126–127